Osteoporosis in Focus

Osteoporosis in Focus

Niall Ferguson

BSc, MSc, MRPharmS

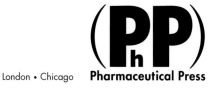

London • Chicago   **Pharmaceutical Press**

Published by the Pharmaceutical Press
Publications division of the Royal Pharmaceutical Society of Great Britain

1 Lambeth High Street, London SE1 7JN, UK
100 South Atkinson Road, Suite 206, Grayslake, IL 60030-7820, USA

© Niall Ferguson 2004

(**P.P**) is a trademark of Pharmaceutical Press

Text design by Barker/Hilsdon, Lyme Regis, Dorset
Typeset by Type Study, Scarborough, North Yorkshire
Printed in Great Britain by TJ International, Padstow, Cornwall

ISBN 0 85369 483 4

A catalogue record for this book is available from the British Library

To the memory of my father, Joseph Watt Ferguson, who sadly was not able to share in my success; but at all times his guidance and support have been my rock.

Contents

Preface

Osteoporosis is a disease that is becoming increasingly talked about in both medical and lay circles as interest develops into why more and more people are suffering from the effects. The expertise for prevention and treatment of osteoporosis is held by a number of different specialists who are thin on the ground and, although they hold many of the answers, they are not freely available to be consulted. It was felt that there was a need to collect together the current knowledge on osteoporosis to satisfy the requirements of a number of different groups of people on various aspects of the disease. Therefore, this book has been written in order to make this information more widely accessible to medics, nurses, pharmacists, other health professionals and interested members of the public.

A wide range of literature has been researched, from recognised textbooks and the most recent clinical studies from journals, in order to amass the clinical knowledge required for this book. The first five chapters look at the disease itself and how it can develop as a result of lifestyle factors. The background and the reason for making clinical interventions are described in Chapter 6. Drug therapy is detailed in the next three chapters, with the future developments laid out in Chapter 11. The issues surrounding patient screening and pharmaceutical care are expanded on in Chapters 12 and 13 respectively. Where possible, the subjects are discussed in detail, in particular drug therapy. Where time has not allowed or the subject aspect is not thought pertinent, then full references have been given for further reading. It is hoped that the layout of the book will enable readers to be selective and at the same time provide them with an informative guide.

At the time of writing, every effort was made to ensure that the most up-to-date information was included, so that the book could act as reference material in a number of different situations. The relentless pace at which new discoveries are made and new developments pioneered makes it impossible to predict future progress, but the guiding principles are there to build on. The book should be consulted in order to obtain both background material for further studies and to provide the basic principles behind the strategies for prevention and treatment.

It is hoped that this book will act as a catalyst for the development of multidisciplinary approaches between a number of health professionals in different spheres, building on the start made in the few collaborative projects that are reported in the text. In this way, osteoporosis awareness amongst the public will be raised, facilitating the identification of the disease at an earlier stage and thus improving the prevention and treatment rates for what is a mainly preventable condition. The aim is to reduce the incidence of fractures and associated patient morbidity, which are not only expensive to treat but also considerably reduce quality of life for a large number of people.

Niall Ferguson
February 2004

Acknowledgements

I would like to acknowledge the help and support of my family in the writing of this book. I would particularly like to mention the role my mother played in her capacity as 'proofreader' and her extensive guidance, for without that support this book might not have been completed. My thanks also to my nearest and dearest for their patience while I was occupied with this task.

About the author

Niall Ferguson obtained a BSc degree in pharmacy in 1982 from Sunderland University and in the following year completed a pre-registration placement in hospital pharmacy. Since qualifying as a pharmacist he has worked extensively in hospital pharmacy in a number of different hospitals.

In 1987 he completed the Clinical Pharmacy Diploma at Aston University followed by the national course in medicines information in 1988. In 1989 Niall, now a clinical tutor, was invited to teach on a course as part of an Oxford regional initiative to become a recognised regional centre for the University of Wales and Institute of Science and Technology (UWIST) Clinical Pharmacy Diploma. A move to Cheshire led to involvement in the initial development of the John Moores University Clinical Pharmacy Diploma, first as part of the management team and subsequently as a clinical tutor. Using advances in computer technology, Niall designed and introduced one of the first electronic databases to record and report clinical interventions and medicines information enquiries. The introduction of competency-based training for the pre-registration pharmacist highlighted the need for a recognised qualification in assessment. This resulted in 1995 in the attainment of the National Vocational Qualification (NVQ) D32–33. In the same year he commenced an MSc degree in clinical pharmacy at Keele University, involving a project on the communication of discharge information on medication from secondary care to primary care. This was completed in 1996.

In 1999, Niall published his first paper on osteoporosis, which looked at treatment of the disease within an orthopaedic unit. In 2000, his paper on drug treatment of osteoporosis was published. In recent years, he has been involved in re-engineering projects in hospital pharmacy with the successful introduction of Patients' Own Drug (POD) and Self Administration of Medicines (SAM) schemes. Niall has also participated in the National/Regional Hip Replacement Re-Engineering Project, which aims to reduce patient stay in hospital to five days.

The author's current interests include the development of medicines management systems, which allow for the use of computer-generated information to be transmitted from secondary care to primary care.

Niall Ferguson is a member of the Royal Pharmaceutical Society of Great Britain (RSPGB).

Abbreviations

ALP	Alkaline phosphatase
BGP	Bone Gla protein
BMD	Bone mineral density
BMU	Bone multicellular unit
COPD	Chronic obstructive pulmonary disease
CSM	Committee on Safety of Medicines
DEXA	Dual-energy X-ray absorptiometry
DNA	Deoxyribonucleic acid
D-Pyr	Deoxypyridinoline
ECF	Extracellular fluid
FSH	Follicle-stimulating hormone
HDL	High-density lipoprotein
HRT	Hormone replacement therapy
LH	Luteinising hormone
MRI	Magnetic resonance imaging
NOS	National Osteoporosis Society
NSAID	Non-steroidal anti-inflammatory drugs
NSF	National Service Framework
OC	Oral contraceptives
Pyr	Pyridinoline
QCT	Quantitative computer tomography
RDA	Recommended daily amount
RNA	Ribonucleic acid
SD	Standard deviation
SERM	Selective oestrogen receptor modulators
SPA	Single-beam photon absorptiometry
SXA	Single-energy X-ray absorptiometry
TRAP	Tartrate-resistant acid phosphatase
TSH	Thyroid-stimulating hormone
WHO	World Health Organization

1

Introduction

The saying 'Old age cometh not alone' is as true as always – it almost always brings with it changes that result in difficulties in health and mobility. However, it is often not until an elderly person suffers a fall and subsequent fracture that the problem of osteoporosis surfaces.

Osteoporosis is a quiet, insidious condition which only manifests itself in later life in the form of a low-impact fracture of the wrist, hip or spine. It is becoming a major clinical problem amongst the ever-increasing numbers of the elderly population in Western countries. In the UK, figures are as high as 200 000 fractures a year, costing the Treasury £1000 million to treat.[1] Worldwide, the number of fractures runs into the millions and is predicted to rise to 6 million within 50 years.

Fortunately, the amount of information that is currently available regarding the causes, diagnosis and management of osteoporosis is also increasing rapidly. This is helping to create a greater understanding of the effects of this clinical problem as realised in the morbidity and immobility caused by related fractures.

Although we are gaining insight into the scale of the problem, which is likely to affect anyone within the general population in time, we have not yet examined the effect on the individual and their quality of life. Over the last ten years, the emphasis in the management of the disease has changed from the mending of the resultant fractures to the discussion of strategies to prevent secondary or even primary fractures. This has led to the development of guidelines by a number of learned bodies, setting standards of management for both the prevention and treatment of osteoporosis. These standards have been put in place to reduce the number of total fractures by early detection of the disease, implementation of preventative treatments and the use of secondary prevention.

In common with a number of disorders, osteoporosis should be viewed as a condition for which 'prevention is better than cure'. Equal emphasis has to be placed both on health promotion to the general population regarding the best methods of prevention and on treatments available to reduce fractures. Prevention must start early in life, preferably before adulthood is attained. Advice should be given on how to maintain a healthy diet and on ensuring that a person's lifestyle contains a reasonable level of load-bearing exercise. The health promotion message needs to be spelled out to each and every generation of the population, as it is never too early or too late for some benefit to be derived.

Treatment options are varied and in some cases complex regimens are employed to maximise benefits from different pathways. Drug therapy for osteoporosis requires careful explanation with regard to how it should be taken, not only to optimise the effects, but also to minimise the possible side-effects. Patients should be given detailed instructions on how to administer the medicines, the usual standard dose, the frequency and timing in relation to food. All these factors will help to maintain patient compliance in the short term. However, to enlist and establish patient cooperation in the long term will require further education in the continuing benefits to be obtained from therapy and, conversely, in the speed with which such advantages will diminish in a very short space of time after the cessation of therapy.

The provision of this type of information from a number of different health professionals, in conjunction with detailed written information from other sources, gives patients a wealth of knowledge. Armed with this information they are then able to take a lead in the management of their disease, knowing that they can obtain further information from either the original source or a particular specialist. This is the informed approach, whereby the patient is given all necessary means to decide on treatment options through the patient-orientated team method.

This collaborative patient care procedure enables patients to take a more active role in the management of their disease; the emphasis is on the patient's quality of life and how this can be improved or maintained with various courses of action, of which drug treatment is only one element, defined as pharmaceutical care. This approach promotes a patient-friendly mode of introduction to medication, minimising clinical interventions for the least disruption in lifestyle, but maximising the value placed on quality of life. On this basis policies are drawn up and discussed between health professionals so that a uniform approach based on the best available evidence from clinical trials is taken.

In order to provide effective patient care, there is a need to weave together all the various strands of therapy into a multidisciplinary approach, thus delivering an all inclusive care package. This book aims to give the reader the background on the reasons why osteoporosis may develop and to show how the condition can be ameliorated with preventative treatment. Treatment consists of drug therapy, the consideration and possible alteration of lifestyle factors and diet changes to produce the best possible outcome. This book aims to set out all the information in a logical manner, presenting the scientific facts along with the clinical aspects of the disease. It will provide a summary of the information available on osteoporosis, as well as its prevention and treatment, with an emphasis on drug therapy and how it can be used both to treat and to prevent the disease. The aim is also to show how the clinical care of the patient is managed by a number of different health professionals.

The knowledge base on osteoporosis is expanding continually on all aspects of clinical care, including length of treatment, new drugs, diagnostic factors and physical aids. While every effort has been made prior to publication to obtain the latest information and check it for accuracy, this may prove to be out of date in the future. This fact should be borne in mind when reading the book, in particular with regard to drug therapy, its indications, doses, frequency, length of treatment, benefits and adverse effects. If in doubt, consult the most recently published information or the manufacturer regarding the specific drug in question for clarification of any point.[2]

Today osteoporosis is one of the foremost diseases afflicting Western society; on the one hand, increasing numbers of the population suffer from it and on the other hand, knowledge both of treatment and of prevention is growing constantly. This means that there is an immense scope for improvement in patient care, particularly in health promotion and pharmaceutical care. The knowledge gained from this publication should enable the reader to develop an enlightened approach to patient care.[3]

References

1. Royal College of Physicians. *Osteoporosis. Clinical Guidelines for Prevention and Treatment.* London: Royal College of Physicians, 1999.
2. Consensus Development Conference; diagnosis, prophylaxis and treatment of osteoporosis. *Am J Med* 1993; 94: 646–650.
3. *Osteoporosis – Are You at Risk?* (leaflet). London: National Osteoporosis Society, 2000.

2

Osteoporosis

Osteoporosis – literally 'porous bones' – has been a known diagnosis since the nineteenth century, when the name was first coined by German pathologists to distinguish it from various other bone diseases. It was redefined in the 1940s, when the condition was stated to be a lack of bone tissue while at the same time the bones remained calcified.[1] However, it is only in recent years that it has gained significance due to the increasing health cost to society. This is a consequence of the ageing population, who are at the greatest risk of developing this degenerative disease, making it the most common metabolic disorder of bone.[2,3]

Definition

Osteoporosis is defined as a progressive systemic skeletal disease, characterised by low bone mass and micro-architectural deterioration of bone tissue, with a consequent increase in bone fragility and susceptibility to fracture, which typically involves the wrist, spine or hip.[2]

This definition relies on the measurement of bone mass, which is a reliable predictor of bone strength, and can be accurately determined by the use of bone mineral density (BMD). The World Health Organization (WHO) has developed a scale based on comparison of a patient's BMD with that of a healthy young adult, known as the T-score, and previous history of a fracture. The scale is divided into four different categories based on the number of standard deviation (SD) units by which the BMD varies from the normal and the presence or absence of a fracture. The divisions in the scale are normal, low bone mass (osteopenia), osteoporosis and established (severe) osteoporosis (see Diagnostic Focus, below).[4]

The WHO classification is a practical means of defining the risk of sustaining a fracture within the white, female, postmenopausal population. Therefore, the criteria have limitations in their practical application, both within this cohort and outside it. This requires further discussion before proceeding further:[5]

DIAGNOSTIC FOCUS

WHO classification of osteoporosis	
Definition	*Criteria*
Normal	A value for BMD within 1 SD of the young adult reference mean
Low bone mass (osteopenia)	A BMD value of more than 1 SD, but less than 2.5 SD below the young adult reference mean
Osteoporosis	BMD greater than 2.5 SD below the young adult reference mean
Established (severe) osteoporosis	BMD more than 2.5 SD below the young adult reference mean plus one or more fragility fractures

- The values for BMD and fracture risk are independent variables that will show a degree of overlap within individuals. The implication of this is that a risk factor can produce a diagnosis where this is a factor that characterises the disease and predisposes a clinical condition. In a similar way, a number of other diseases can be assessed by a quantifiable risk but not necessarily diagnosed. Furthermore, the risk factor is distributed throughout the whole population, leading to an arbitrary cut-off point that will create a false impression of banding of individuals into the separate categories. The consequence of this is that individuals at the extreme limit of each category may be over- or under-treated. Interpretation of these facts by health care professionals is critical in determining the correct diagnosis and subsequent treatment.

- The classification of the criteria is based on data collated from epidemiological studies on white postmenopausal women. Therefore, this has to be taken into consideration when looking at other cohorts of the population, such as men, other ethnic groups and premenopausal women. It has been shown that the risk of fracture in men is lower than that predicted by BMD T-score. Similarly, in young individuals with corticosteroid-induced osteoporosis, the critical BMD is −1.5 T-score rather than the −2.5 T-score derived from the WHO classification.

- The values obtained were identified using dual-energy X-ray absorptiometry (DEXA) on the axial skeleton. If different diagnostic systems are used, for instance ultrasound, then these techniques must be validated separately before they can be applied to the same definitions and risk factors.

- It is known that the BMD does not give a complete picture of the strength of the bone because this is dependent on the ratio of trabecular bone to cortical bone. Either more information is required on the make-up of the bone to assess its quality from biochemical changes from bone turnover, or physical changes must be identified by ultrasound or direct X-rays.

- There may be other reasons for a low BMD, such as osteomalacia, hyperparathyroidism or a combination of the two. These differential diagnoses should be excluded by biochemical assessment because they are more responsive to specific treatment than advanced osteoporosis.
- Although BMD is a reputable predictor of risk of fracture, it is not the only one; particularly in the elderly population, the propensity to fall can be just as important. In such cases the risk of a fall because of neuromuscular abnormalities, postural hypotension, poor vision, cognitive dysfunction or drug-induced adverse effects can be important.
- The divisions within the WHO classification scale should be used as a guide to aid treatment, not an absolute indication. The third and fourth divisions require clinical intervention, unless the patient has an overriding condition leading to terminal care. The second division is more problematical because the decision to intervene should be made on a case-by-case basis, whereas the first division is normal.

Concern about the limitations of the WHO guidelines has led to the standard setting bodies recommending that the guidelines be used in the context of a case-finding strategy.

Physiological background

Having defined the condition of osteoporosis and all its variations, some attention will now be given to describing normal bone physiology and how it performs everyday functions. Having attempted this, the abnormal picture as seen in osteoporosis will become more apparent and more easily understood.

Bone structure

There are 206 bones within the human skeleton, which itself is split into two main parts: the axial, consisting of the head and the trunk, and the appendicular, which relates to the limbs. The skeleton is a connective tissue, responsible for providing support to the body within a rigid framework. Therefore, the skeleton not only provides the shape of the body, protecting the vital organs, but it also gives the body strength through the reinforced matrix of fibres embedded in minerals that make up the composition of the bone.

Although bone appears to be a solid, inert structure, it is, in fact a dynamic system carrying out a great deal of metabolic activity, which is subject to and modified by a number of factors. Throughout the growing period, the shape of the bone remains resistant to force; if broken, a bone will repair itself to near normal structure. Bone also acts as an ion reservoir, containing over 99% of the body's calcium. This is a vital role within the body.[6]

Architecture of bone

Bones come in various shapes and sizes, but can be divided into two main categories: tubular and flat. The main role of tubular bones is to bear weight and, in order to carry out this function, they are constructed with a dense outer surface of compact (or cortical) bone and a central region or medulla, which comprises narrow plates called trabeculae. The trabecular bone acts as a framework that strengthens the outer casing, enabling it to withstand the everyday strains and stresses caused by daily physical activity. This conformation gives tubular bone maximum strength for minimum weight. The ratio between inner trabecular bone and outer cortical bone varies throughout the skeleton, the determining factor being the force to which the bone is subjected by compression and turning. For example, the appendicular skeleton consists of 20% trabecular bone and 80% cortical bone, whereas the ratio is 50:50 in the spine and hip. In the spaces within the central core of the bone lies the bone marrow, which is in close proximity to cells producing blood cells. This colours the bone marrow red in the early years, although it changes to yellow as fat is deposited throughout adult life.

A tubular bone is made up of a central shaft, known as the diaphysis, with a growing portion called the metaphysis, and at either end are the epiphyses, surrounded by articular cartilage. The bone grows by converting the existing cartilage material into bone by the infiltration of collagen fibres, followed by the deposition of polysaccharide and calcium; this process is known as endochondral ossification because it is carried out within the cartilage. The ossification begins in the centre and then moves towards the ends of the bone; furthermore, in most tubular bones there is a secondary site of ossification, which is located at the ends of the bones, in the epiphyses. Endochondral ossification continues throughout the growth period and the cartilaginous zone exists between the two ossification centres until growth ceases, when the cartilaginous area is completely infiltrated and the remains become the articulating surface of the bone.

The bone grows in length from the metaphysis growth area and increases in girth by deposition underneath the dense outer layer of the bone, which is known as the periosteum. At the same time, the outer layer of the bone marrow, the endosteum, is resorbing bone, which results in the expansion of the bone marrow cavity.

The growth cartilage consists of three layers: the proliferating zone, the matrix and the calcification zone of the matrix. The chondrocyte cells of the cartilage move through these three layers, commencing in the proliferating zone and moving on to aid the formation of the matrix beneath. In becoming part of the matrix, the cells develop Golgi apparatus and large spaces, called cisternae, form in the endoplasmic reticulum. This is a normal characteristic of secretory cells. The cells then begin to enlarge within the matrix, compressing it, prior to the gradual deposition of calcium within the cells. This is the progression to bone. Stage one is the initial mineralisation of the matrix, then the mineral is resorbed by the osteoclasts, and finally new bone is formed by the osteoblasts. This is the process by which bone grows, with the progression of the cartilage leaving bone behind it, until the bone reaches maturity, when proliferation ceases; the growth plate then becomes ossified and fuses with the epiphyses.

In the fully developed bone, 80% by weight is made up of compact bone, which not only comprises the outer surface, but is mostly found in shafts within the tubular bone. The compact bone consists of thin concentric bands called lamellae, which surround a central canal called the Haversian system. These canals run longitudinally through the bone, interconnected by small narrow channels known as canaliculi, to spaces called lacunae, containing osteocytes. These spaces and tubules with the network of channels form a communication network, which allows nutrients and fluid to flow freely throughout the bone. The network is created as the bone is formed, ensuring that all parts of the bone remain within easy access of essential nutrition and in communication via humoral fluid. In particular, it is vital that the central core or marrow has access to nutrition in order to maintain activity by constantly renewing tissue at the end of its life cycle.

Trabecular bone is a rigid framework of mineralised bone that is present in each vertebra and in the epiphyses of the long bones. Although trabecular bone makes up only 20% of the total bone mass, it contributes most to bone strength. The trabeculae are present to ensure that the stresses and strains placed upon bone during weight-bearing exercise and muscle activity are withstood. The number, size and distribution of trabeculae is dependent on the type of force that a particular bone will be required to withstand. In comparison with the more sedentary compact bone, the trabecular bone is the most active part of the skeleton, with a high turnover of trabecular cells, and is provided with a plentiful blood supply. The trabecular bone has the greatest surface area and the highest level of metabolism of all of the sections of the bone. If there is any reduction in mobility and thus activity, the trabecular bone is the part that is most affected.[6,7]

Cellular bone

Bone consists of a number of different types of cells, which are present over the surface of the bone and also in the internal cavities, called lacunae, of the mineralised section of the matrix. These cells are mostly either osteoblasts or osteoclasts; the only other cells present are osteo-cytes and lining cells, which are thought to be inactive osteoblasts.

Osteoblasts

These are the bone-forming cells; they synthesise the bone matrix and produce the consequent mineralisation. Originating from the connective tissue or stroma stem cells, osteoblasts are shaped like cubes and form a single layer attached to the internal surfaces of the bone. The cellular contents of osteoblasts include large amounts of endoplasmic reticulum, to which large vesicles known as the Golgi apparatus are connected; this is characteristic of a secretory cell. Mitochondria are evident in the cyto-plasm covered with a mineral deposit; the deposit is granular in shape, consisting of calcium, phosphate, a trace of magnesium and organic matter. The mitochondria are able to actively concentrate the calcium from the cell cytoplasm into these granules, thus regulating calcium levels within the cell. Each osteoblast has numerous connections with its neighbours through small channels called microtubules, which permit the passage of fluids and nutrients necessary for the survival of that cell. The cube-like shape of the osteoblast is maintained by an internal frame-work of microfilaments, which give the cell mobility and contractility.

The osteoblast cell forms bone matrix by synthesising and secreting both collagen and mucopolysaccharides. The matrix is produced as a thin layer between the calcified bone and the osteoblast prior to being mineralised. Osteoblasts are also known to synthesise a number of other proteins, such as collagenase, prostaglandin E_2, osteocalcin and osteonectin. There are also receptors for a variety of calcium-regulating substances, including parathyroid hormone, vitamin D, prostaglandin E_2 and glucocorticoids.

As the osteoblast matures through its life cycle, the matrix vesicles are shed, thus permitting mineralisation of the tissue as inhibition to calcification is lost.

Osteoclasts

Osteoclasts are large, multinucleated cells that play an active role in bone resorption. They are derived from a haematopoietic stem cell line, which itself is derived from a phagocytic cell line, and thus possess the properties of both. Produced by the coming together of mononucleated cells to form cells with anything from two to 200 nuclei, osteoclasts are found on the surface of the bone, close to the sites of resorbed bone, where they cause concave depressions, known as Howship's lacunae. The osteoclasts are attached to the bone by microvilli, which actively resorb bone. Each cell controls its own area of bone, separate from other cells and close to a site of bone mineralisation.

Osteoclasts are not active all the time, but are activated by various humoral substances such as parathyroid hormone, vitamin D or prostaglandin. They secrete substances that break down the bone, for example citrates; this causes a demineralisation of the bone and the removal of the calcium. Collagenase is also released, which breaks down the surrounding protein of the bone; the protein molecular and calcium ions extracted are then stored in numerous cavities called vacuoles and vesicles.

This is the method by which osteoclasts remodel the bone, in opposition to osteoblasts. Osteoclasts are far more efficient and are far fewer in number than osteoblasts.

Osteocytes

At first glance, a variation on the osteoblast, the osteocyte does not seem to have a function in bone, and remains relatively inactive. Osteocytes live on the surface of the bone and are enveloped by the lacunae cavities within the mineralised bone; the cells themselves are mineralised once they have been encased in the osteoid protein. The osteocyte has all the characteristics of the osteoblast, containing a large amount of endoplasmic reticulum, Golgi bodies and many mitochondria in the cytoplasm of the cell. The difference between the osteoblast and the osteocyte is that the latter has a number of channels, both in the cytoplasm and at the interface of the individual cells; this permits ease of transfer of nutrients and fluid to the numerous cells, both osteocytes and osteoblasts.

Osteocytes, although mainly dormant, are activated by the influence of the calcium-modulating hormones parathyroid and calcitonin; this is important as the osteocytes exert a calcium-regulatory effect.

Osteoblasts, osteoclasts and osteocytes are the main types of functional cells that constitute bone (see Bone Focus, below), but bone also contains a number of structures made up of supportive and connecting tissues. The bone matrix is one such structure. This consists of collagen and mineralised mucopolysaccharides, which provide strength and rigidity to bone and allow the bone to sustain the normal forces associated with movement. The strength of the bone stems from the manner in which the collagen and mineral are put together and the specific pattern of the collagen fibres. This collagen network within the bone makes up 65% of the organic component of bone. Other organic components include non-cellular proteins, proteoglycans and lipids, which are thought to be important in fracture repair.

The collagen within bone derives from either fibroblasts or osteoblasts as a helical structure of three long polypeptide chains, known as alpha chains. This form of collagen is specific to bone, and its synthesis is controlled by gene material from the cell's deoxyribonucleic acid (DNA).

Bone collagen is the only form of collagen within the body that is mineralised and it interacts with a number of other tissue components, namely proteoglycans, glycoproteins and minerals, which are specific to bone. This creates a problem when it has to be renewed, because the mineral component, hydroxyapatite, must be removed before the collagen can be broken down by the collagenase enzymes into peptides and amino acids, to be excreted via the kidney.

Proteoglycan is a mucopolysaccharide consisting of a polypeptide centre with a number of polysaccharide side-chains made up of disaccharide units connected to the polypeptide by a link protein. This produces a molecule with a net negative charge, which emits a strong

BONE FOCUS

Bone cells	Function
Osteoblasts	Control bone formation
Osteoclasts	Control bone resorption
Osteocytes	Permit calcium uptake into bone

attraction to cations. These bind strongly and are available for the synthesis of collagen, particularly at the mineralisation stage.

A similar mucopolysaccharide is glycoprotein, which again is composed of a polypeptide in the centre of the molecule; in this case, however, the side-chains are formed of a number of different monosaccharide molecules. This causes the glycoprotein molecule to be straighter with less bulk, because of the shorter side-chains.

Two other proteins that are present in bone and that are manufactured by the osteoblasts are osteocalcin and osteonectin. These both bind with calcium and are involved with the deposition of calcium in collagen. The levels of these proteins are increased when bone turnover is occurring and when there is heightened osteoblast activity. During mineralisation, it is the function of these proteins to facilitate the penetration of the hydroxyapatite molecule into the bone matrix.[6,7]

Bone mineral

The mineralisation of the bone matrix is responsible for the mineral content of bone, which in the mature state consists of hydroxyapatite derived from amorphous calcium phosphate or octacalcium phosphate. The most abundant cation in bone is calcium, closely followed by magnesium. There are also traces of sodium and fluoride, which are essential; if either of these two elements is lacking, then any bone formed will be defective.

There is approximately 1.2 kg of calcium in the adult human skeleton, which is 99.9% of the body's total content. Although calcium is present in a number of tissues, where it is essential for vital functions, the content in blood is closely controlled by biofeedback mechanisms involving the parathyroid hormone. In fact, calcium is in dynamic equilibrium in blood, where it is free. In protein, the calcium is bound, but in bone it exists as hydroxyapatite.

Phosphorus is the second most prevalent element in the bone and, like calcium, the content is kept in check between bone and other tissues in the body. However phosphorus is not controlled as rigidly as calcium. Phosphorus is also subject to the influence of the parathyroid hormone and if there is an excess of the parathyroid hormone then an increasing amount of phosphate is excreted in the urine. If this condition persists then phosphorus is mobilised from bone to be excreted in the urine by an increased resorption of calcium and phosphate. As a temporary measure to combat the loss of phosphate in this situation, aluminium may be given, which binds the phosphate in the gastrointestinal tract.

This will control the loss of phosphate for a time, although eventually the release of phosphorus from bone will recommence.

Hydroxyapatite is an inorganic compound that contains calcium both as a phosphate and a hydroxide, with the chemical formula $3Ca_3(PO_4)_2Ca(OH)_2$. It takes the shape of amorphous crystals, which usually form outside the cell, where they are combined with procollagen fibrils to produce a mineralised collagen. Crystals of hydroxyapatite are arranged in a specific pattern on the collagen fibres, where they are bound tightly to a link protein. Once the hydroxyapatite crystals have begun to attach themselves to the collagen, this process continues over a number of days, effecting mineralisation and eventually leading to the development of mature bone.

Bone formation

Bone is an important structure in the body and it is because of this that it is present at an early stage in the development. It is clearly visible in the fetus at around the 26th week of gestation. At this stage, the long bones have formed into the relative size and shape seen in a fully developed infant; furthermore, the skeleton structure is also present, prior to the process of mineralisation occurring.

Towards the end of pregnancy, the skeleton of the fetus becomes mineralised, using elements taken from the mother. This results in a large amount of calcium being drained from the mother – generally up to 200 mg daily. If the mother does not obtain a high level of calcium from her daily diet to replace this, either she will lose calcium from her skeleton or else the fetus will be deprived.

Once the infant is born, the bone continues its growth for approximately the next 20 years, with a growth spurt some time in the teenage years. This is followed by a period of consolidation when, in the third decade, the level of bone reaches its peak. This is first attained by the trabecular bone and succeeded by the cortical bone.

The peak level to which a skeleton can develop is dictated by genetic inheritance, but an individual's attainment of his or her peak level is influenced by environment and growth factors. These factors determine the manner in which the skeleton is modelled from the raw materials and range from the diet to the physical demands made upon the bone by the daily wear and tear of everyday life. If, in a population, any of these factors are enhanced, for example by a widespread increase of calcium in the diet, the people will benefit from an increase in bone mass and a general growth in stature will be observed.

Remodelling

As we have discussed, bone is not a static system, but a dynamic one, continually turning over and repairing itself, making good all the damage incurred from the mechanical stresses and strains to which it is subject during daily living. This process is known as remodelling and is carried out within a cycle of bone formation and bone resorption (see Bone Focus, below). These two opposing processes appear to be activated at variable rates, with no one specific factor predicting or determining which process will be dominant in either the increases or the decreases of bone mass.

The remodelling of compact bone is instigated by the osteoclasts, which are at the forefront of resorption of bone. The osteoclasts form a cone shape and, by cutting into older mineralised bone, create a cavity. This new cavity develops into a Haversian system with the osteoblast, which being at some distance from the resorption process, starts producing new cells that eventually develop into new mineralised bone tissue. A similar process occurs in trabecular bone, where the osteoclasts create new cavities, with the osteoblast renewing the bone; however this activity proceeds at a much faster rate in the trabecular bone than in the compact bone. These localised 'teams' of osteoblasts and osteoclasts by which bone renews itself are called bone multicellular units (BMUs).

BMUs, contained within the bone, generally work in conjunction and counterbalance one another, ensuring that bone turnover and bone mass remain more or less the same. However, if the system is thrown out of balance and a net bone loss occurs, an increase in the size and number of Haversian canals occurs. The outcome of this malfunction is an increase in the porosity of the compact bone and a loss of trabeculae from trabecular bone and a consequent rise in the volume of splinters or spicules.

BONE FOCUS

Processes in bone	
Bone formation	Development of new bone controlled by osteoblasts
Bone resorption	The removal of bone by osteoclasts
Bone remodelling	The regeneration of bone, repairing microfractures
Bone turnover	The combination of bone resorption and formation

Repair

The remodelling process is the means by which minute bone damage is repaired on a continuous basis. However, while bone damage increases with age, the remodelling process does not keep pace; therefore, with the loss of the repair mechanism, the bone begins to lose strength and as the amount of damage increases the ability to repair diminishes.

When the fracture of a normal bone occurs, the area of fracture fills with granulation tissue, which is composed of capillaries, fibroblasts and progenitor cells. The progenitor cells rapidly produce osteoblasts, which begin the process of repair by synthesising bone matrix and commencing mineralisation. This produces bone that is irregular in comparison with the surrounding bone. This condition is rectified over the next two to four years, until the pattern of the new bone is the same as that of the existing bone. Remodelling of the bone ensures that the fracture becomes completely repaired, presenting a seamless join with the original bone. A fracture in an osteoporotic bone will be repaired in the normal manner, but in cases of osteomalacia an incomplete repair is made because of the abnormal remodelling.

Bone growth

Remodelling and bone growth are controlled by a number of factors. These are primarily: the amount of raw material available, the effect of mechanical forces on the bone, and systemic and local growth factors. Bone growth, as explained earlier, occurs as a result of the remodelling and resorption processes. These are influenced by systemic factors, since it is vital that all bones grow at the same rate in order to maintain the symmetry of the body. This is in contrast to bone strength, which tends to be controlled by local factors because of the particular stresses and strains from usual body activity. In the mature bone, once growth has been completed the dual processes of formation and resorption are governed by local factors. However, these are occasionally overridden by a systemic effect, for instance if loss of oestrogen has occurred.

While attempting to elucidate the method by which bone grows, it has been discovered that the process is a complicated one and it has not yet been fully revealed. Bone growth takes place at a number of levels, namely molecular, cellular, tissue and organ. Under the influence of controlling hormones, the DNA and messenger RNA of the collagen gene operate at the molecular level to synthesise new collagen. At the cellular level the osteoblasts and osteoclasts appear to operate in conjunction with each other, but it is not yet clear exactly how they interact.[6,7]

Calcium-controlling hormones

The use of calcium in the mineral metabolism of bone is controlled by three hormones: calcitonin, parathyroid hormone and vitamin D (see Controlling Factor Focus, below).

Calcitonin is a polypeptide hormone originating in the C cells of the thyroid gland. It consists of a sequence of 32 amino acids, which is released as a precursor together with an attached additional peptide called katacalcin, which possesses calcium-controlling properties.[8]

Calcitonin is secreted in response to a high calcium serum level and is diminished in the presence of a low calcium serum level; 1,25-dihydroxyvitamin D (calcitriol) also acts as a stimulant to calcitonin secretion. The effects of calcitonin are believed to be used to counteract a short-term elevation of calcium in the body brought about by a high dietary intake of calcium which, if not rectified, would lead to hyper-calcaemia and hypercalciuria. Although, calcitonin does inhibit osteo-clast bone resorption, thus preventing calcium release from bone, calcitonin does not greatly affect the calcium serum level because of the more profound effect of the other calcium-regulating hormones. The other known effect of calcitonin is that it increases activity of the renal enzyme 1-α-hydroxylase, which increases the production of 1,25-dihydroxyvitamin D.

Parathyroid hormone is the most important influence on the control of plasma calcium. This hormone is synthesised in the chief cells of the parathyroid gland and is a polypeptide of 84 amino acids, of which only 34 amino acids of the terminal fragment make up the active part of the hormone. When calcium serum levels are low, parathyroid hormone is secreted, mobilising calcium from bone, increasing absorp-tion of calcium from the intestine and reducing loss of calcium through the kidney. Parathyroid hormone has a direct effect on the osteoclasts

CONTROLLING FACTOR FOCUS

Calcium-regulating hormones

Calcitonin – increases calcium uptake into cells including bone

Parathyroid hormone – increases calcium levels in circulation by mobilising calcium from bone

Vitamin D – increases the level of calcium in the body through improved absorption by altering their morphology in order to increase bone resorption. In the kidney, parathyroid hormone increases calcium resorption, at the same time reducing phosphate resorption; this produces an increase in calcium but a reduction in calcium phosphate, allowing ready supply of calcium for use in bone mineral. Parathyroid hormone also increases synthesis of 1,25-dihydroxyvitamin D in the kidney, which increases absorption of calcium from the intestine.

The third calcium-controlling hormone, vitamin D, is obtained from either diet or exposure to sunlight. It needs to be metabolised in the liver and then in the kidney before it is activated to the active di-hydroxy form. This metabolite of vitamin D has an effect on the gastro-intestinal tract, via which it increases absorption of calcium and phosphate. The ultimate effect of all this activity on the bone is to stimulate bone resorption and inhibit collagen synthesis.

There are also systemic hormones that have a direct effect on bone and that are responsible for controlling bone growth and thus determining bone mass (see Controlling Factor Focus, below). Glucocorticoids at normal physiological levels have an important effect on bone growth by increasing collagen synthesis. If doses of glucocorticoids that are greater than physiological levels are administered, then an opposite effect to the one just described is obtained: bone growth is reduced and a decrease in bone mass ensues. Therefore, it can be observed that the effect produced by the administration of glucocorticoids is solely dependent on the dose. A dose greater than the physiological level can bring about an inhibitory effect on bone growth.

Growth hormone, as the name suggests, has a beneficial effect on bone growth, probably by activating somatomedin synthesis, which directly enhances collagen and non-collagen protein synthesis.

CONTROLLING FACTOR FOCUS

Systemic hormones that regulate bone
Growth hormone
Glucocorticoids
Insulin
Sex hormones
Somatomedins
Levothyroxine (thyroxine)

Insulin is another hormone whose effect on bone growth is dependent on its concentration. At low levels, as seen in the deficiency disease diabetes mellitus, insulin reduces bone growth by creating a condition of poor nutrition. This in turn leads to a lack of essential nutrients. In the non-diabetic individual, insulin increases collagen synthesis by improving nutrition.

The sex hormones have a considerable effect on bone growth and the maintenance of bone mass. Oestrogen is known to promote bone growth in the child and to maintain bone mass in the adult; if there is a deficiency of oestrogen, then bone growth will be reduced in the child and bone mass is lost in the adult. Androgens are important in the male and are thought to be responsible for the growth spurt seen in adolescent boys.[6]

Local bone growth

A number of other bone growth factors can be detected in biological fluids in or around bone. The influence of these factors ranges from new bone formation to the development of bone from cartilage, bone matrix synthesis, mineralisation and resorption.

Prostaglandin E_2 seems to be important in the linking of osteoblast and osteoclast activity. At low concentrations, prostaglandin promotes bone growth through an increase in osteoblast activity; at high concentrations the osteoclast activity is increased, leading to osteolysis and hypercalcaemia, as is often seen in neoplastic conditions.

Various cytokines help both in bone formation and bone resorption, but the overall effect is to inhibit bone formation by aiding the release of enzymes that break down bone and collagen. These cytokines include interleukin 1, tumour necrosis factor, lymphotoxin and colony-stimulating factors.

Calcium and phosphate are necessary for bone formation and are maintained in the body by a number of hormones. If there is a deficiency of calcium then resorption will be increased in order to release calcium into the circulation to maintain concentrations both in and around cells. If phosphate is lacking then mineralisation will be decreased, as phosphate is important in regulating bone metabolism.[9]

Epidemiology

Epidemiology is defined as the study of the occurrence, distribution and control of a disease within the population. Originally applied only to infectious diseases, it is now used equally in relation to non-infectious diseases.[10] The information gathered from the study of the epidemiology provides public authorities with some foreknowledge of the prevalence of a disease and allows plans to be put in place for the marshalling of resources for either treatment or prevention.

The problem with osteoporosis is that it can be present in a patient for many years without any apparent consequences, either as symptoms or as a medical condition that would prompt the patient to seek medical advice.

The one event that does indicate the possible presence of osteoporosis is the occurrence of a fracture, which, if investigated, will in certain circumstances reveal the presence of osteoporosis. The incidence of fractures has a bimodal distribution, peaking in the teenage years and in people over 50 years old. Between these two age groups, there is a steady decline before the incidence of fractures rises, notably in the elderly and continues to increase with age. In the young, fractures tend to be of the long bones, and usually occur as a result of accidents either in sports or related to road traffic. These accidental fractures are more common in boys than in girls, whereas in the elderly, women have a higher incidence of fracture than men.

Common fractures in later life are vertebral, proximal humerus, proximal femur, distal forearm, pelvis and colles, particularly in women in their late forties. In women in their fifties, the incidence of vertebral fracture increases rapidly, with a significant number of these comprising crush fractures. It is not until people are over 70 that the fracture of the proximal femur becomes the most frequent fracture. As a person ages, the change in the site of fracture is probably related to the loss of cortical and trabecular bone at these specific locations.

Fractures that occur in elderly patients have consequences on their quality of life, resulting in morbidity and even in mortality. Fracture of the femur can affect mobility and the ability of a person to cope independently; this puts an extra burden on either their family or the state. A vertebral fracture will at the least cause pain, leading to the use of analgesics for a long or short period. This type of fracture can also result in loss of height.

The description, given above, of a loss of bone mass occurring with increasing age and resulting in a related fracture, would appear to indicate that it would be possible to predict the likelihood of an individual sustaining a fracture based on their age. This does have some validity, but it is not definitive as there appears to be the necessity for an initiating event to take place before a fracture is sustained. This could be a simple fall and the cause of the fall could be determined by a number of factors unrelated to the patient's bone mass.

A patient's susceptibility to a fracture related to bone mass is more accurately gauged by assessing the strength of the bone. The content of the bone, namely the relative amounts of cortical and trabecular bone, is the factor by which the strength of the bone is determined. The manner in which the bone mass has been lost and from which area of the bone indicates the amount of strength that has been lost. It is the trabecular bone that is the most important in this respect, as it permits the bone to withstand external forces, thus preventing fracture. Trabecular bone is lost uniformly: in the areas where it is thinnest it may be lost altogether; further weakening occurs when there is a lack of repair to microfractures from impaired healing, due to the lack of the normal repair function.[11]

The menopause

Osteoporosis has long been considered a disease of postmenopausal women, but it is not exclusively so. More recently it has been recognised in men as a consequence of the increase in the ageing population. Although the condition develops throughout life, the first signs of the disease do not appear until later life. In women, this can be from the age of 45, but the greatest incidence is seen between the ages of 60 and 80 years in both sexes.

Because diagnosis of osteoporosis is normally only made following a fracture, the incidence of the disease is difficult to determine. It is easier to quantify the risk of a fracture based on the actual fracture rate within the known population. As a result, any values produced will always be an estimate of the true incidence.

The lifetime risk of a fracture in a white woman is thought to be in the region of 30–40%, whereas the estimated figure in men is between 6 and 11%. The incidence increases with age between the ages of 60 and 80 years, and there appears to be a five-year gap between the sexes whereby a 75-year-old woman has the same incidence of fracture as an 80-year-old man.

A first fracture will increase the likelihood of a second fracture of the hip or spine by as much as 20-fold, and the annual incidence of second hip fracture is 2.2% in women and 1.5% in men. These figures account for the higher hospital bed occupancy (by women) caused by osteoporosis than most common diseases. The significance of the problem is highlighted by the fact that 20% of hip fracture patients will die in the first year and more than 50% fail to regain their full functional mobility to lead an independent life.[12]

Signs and symptoms

Initially a patient will have no symptoms before presenting with a low-grade impact fracture of the wrist or hip; this will be the first sign of any underlying problem. The severity of the condition at presentation will dictate whether there are any further symptoms. Similarly, the site of the fracture and the degree of complication will affect the severity and number of different symptoms.

Although a hip or wrist fracture will be painful at presentation, once it has healed the patient will generally be pain free. If there are any complications with healing, the patient may remain in pain until the fracture has been successfully restored. In the hip this may remain a constant problem, leading to limited or no mobility.

If the presenting fracture is a compression fracture of the spine, this will not only cause acute pain at onset but may also, depending on the severity, lead to further complications. A spinal compression fracture may put pressure on the spinal column, which contains numerous nerve pathways. This will lead to neuropathic pain that can be spontaneous and extreme, arising from low threshold stimuli or unusual stimuli due to the heightened response to pain. This may cause the patient to become cautious in attempting any movement, to prevent the generation of further pain. Posture may change as the patient adopts a stance in which pain is reduced. Not knowing when the next bout of pain may commence may cause the patient to feel a lack of confidence, leading to reduced mobility, insecurity and anxiety, which can in turn cause depression. The initial vertebral fracture induces a change in the architecture of the spine, as the vertebrae change position and alignment. This may be noticed as a slight curvature of the spine; further vertebral fractures will emphasise the curvature of the spine, producing a change in posture, which if marked, can affect respiration.[3]

Types of conditions

Osteoporosis can be classified into two different categories: primary (idiopathic), in which there are no apparent causal factors, and secondary when a specific cause is isolated. This classification can be misleading as the distinguishing factors are artificial; often there are a number of predisposing factors and no one specific diagnosis can be isolated.

These two categories have been further distinguished by detailing the more specific diagnostic factors as listed in the Diagnostic Focus below.

DIAGNOSTIC FOCUS

Classification of osteoporosis

Diagnosis	Description	Examples
Primary osteoporosis	Lack of oestrogen as part of the natural ageing process	Postmenopausal osteoporosis (type I), vertebral crush fracture syndrome Senile osteoporosis (type II), fracture of the proximal femur
	In children with normal gonadal function	Idiopathic osteoporosis
	In adolescents with normal gonadal function	Juvenile osteoporosis
Endocrine osteoporosis	Calcium and vitamin D absorption affected by endocrine malfunction	Hyperparathyroidism Cushing's syndrome Hyperthyroidism Hypogonadism Diabetes mellitus
Nutritional osteoporosis	Lack of dietary calcium and vitamin D	Scurvy Malnutrition Calcium deficiency Malabsorption
Secondary osteoporosis	Calcium and vitamin D absorption and metabolism disrupted by other conditions	Alcoholism Liver disease Renal disease
Haematopoietic osteoporosis	Breakdown of bone by plasmacytomas	Myeloma Lymphoma Leukaemia Mast cell disease Thalassaemia
Congenital osteoporosis		Osteogenesis imperfecta Homocystinuria
Osteomalacia	Softening of bone due to deficiency of calcium and vitamin D	Nutritional Malabsorptive Renal Vitamin D resistance caused by anticonvulsant drugs (e.g. phenytoin, carbamazepine)

Primary osteoporosis can be subdivided into two further sections: type I or vertebral crush fracture syndrome, which is generally seen in women about ten years after the menopause, and type II or senile and involutional osteoporosis, which is generally see in older patients with fracture neck of femur.

Vertebral crush fracture syndrome usually presents as acute onset of back pain, which, following X-ray investigation, shows one or two fractures, usually without any trauma. Occasionally chronic back pain can be a manifestation of compressed vertebrae; in this case, height loss coupled with some deformity can be present, but without pain.

Another form of primary osteoporosis is the relatively rare disorder of juvenile osteoporosis. This develops at the time of the growth spurt during puberty and is characterised by an unexplained lack of consolidation of bone and consequently strength. Juvenile osteoporosis may lead to frequent fractures.

Secondary osteoporosis can resemble the clinical picture of primary osteoporosis. The differences are often only detected at cell level when histological examination is carried out. The histology can be specific to the particular causative factor, for instance osteitis fibrosa cystica in hyperparathyroidism and hyperthyroidism, abnormal collagen patterns in osteogenesis imperfecta, characteristic abnormal cells in myeloma and mastocytoma.

In order to consider a diagnosis of osteoporosis, a full medical history should be sought to identify all possible risk factors likely to be involved, so that management of the condition can be optimised. Once the possible risk factors have been evaluated then the strategy for management can be implemented, highlighting the areas giving the greatest benefit with the least disruption to lifestyle.

There are a number of conditions related to osteoporosis, which will be considered below. But first it is important to differentiate between the terms osteoporosis, osteopenia and osteomalacia. Osteopenia is the change in biochemical profile showing a lowering of blood calcium which, if uncorrected, will lead to osteoporosis; osteomalacia is a softening of bones caused by an inability to form the correct bone structure.[3,5]

Differential diagnosis

In the definition of osteoporosis, bone changes are identified without specifying the possible cause. However, prior to the commencement of any treatment it is essential to determine the underlying cause so that appropriate therapy can be selected. There are a few conditions that are reversible and are not progressive and if therapy commences without knowledge of the cause of the osteoporosis, then further deterioration may continue despite the treatment.

In order to be certain that a low BMD is the result of loss of bone structure, some straightforward biochemical tests should be undertaken, in particular measurement of parathyroid hormone to exclude hyper-parathyroidism. If this is detected then restorative treatment should be given prior to any further measurements of BMD.

If no apparent cause can be found for the osteoporosis, either from lifestyle factors or external causes, and the patient has abnormal bone biochemical markers, then a bone biopsy should be performed to eliminate osteomalacia.[5]

References

1. Albright F, Smith P H, Richardson A M. Postmenopausal osteoporosis. Its clinical features. *JAMA* 1941; **116**: 2465–2474.

2. Consensus Development Conference; diagnosis, prophylaxis and treatment of osteoporosis. *Am J Med* 1993; **94**: 646–650.

3. Kanis J A. *Osteoporosis*. Oxford: Blackwell Science, 1996.

4. World Health Organization. Assessment of fracture risk and its application to screening for postmenopausal osteoporosis. *World Health Organ Tech Rep Ser* 1994; No. 843.

5. South African Medical Association – Osteoporosis Working Group. Osteo-porosis clinical guideline. *S Afr Med J* 2000; **90**: 907–944.

6. Woolf A D, Dixon A S. *Osteoporosis: a Clinical Guide*. London: Martin Dunitz, 1988.

7. Clegg C P, Clegg A G. *Biology of the Mammal*. Oxford: Heinemann Medical Books, 1975.

8. Hillyard C J, Myers C, Abeyasekera G, Stevvensvenson JC, Craig RK, MacIntyre I. Katacalcin. *Lancet* 1983; **2**: 846–848.

9. Canalis E. Local bone growth factors. *Calcif Tissue Int* 1984; **36**: 632–634.

10. *Oxford Medical Dictionary*. Oxford: Oxford University Press, 1998.

11. Royal College of Physicians. *Osteoporosis. Clinical Guidelines for Prevention and Treatment*. London: Royal College of Physicians, 1999.

12. Common issues in osteoporosis. *MeReC Bull* 2001; **12**(2): 5–8.

3

Prevention of osteoporosis

In the natural process of ageing it is inevitable that the human body will suffer some bone loss in the long term, and that this loss will occur over a period of years. It is necessary, therefore, to consider putting into practice some method of reducing or arresting this process in order that elderly people can survive into old age without being unduly troubled by the onset of osteoporosis. The level of intervention needed for each person will be different and will be characterised and determined by the different factors of each case. The main aim is to prevent excessive loss of bone mass. To this end, the section of the population most at risk needs to be selected and targeted with preventative measures.

The benchmark in the prevention of osteoporosis is based on an individual's peak bone mass, as achieved in early adult life, and the rate of loss occurring during later life. It follows, therefore, that prevention can be divided into a number of phases depending on the age of the individual. In the earlier stages of life, prevention is based on ensuring that the optimum peak bone mass is gained, whereas in later life the aim is to reduce bone mass loss in order to prevent the onset of osteoporosis.

The type of prevention just described is known as primary prevention, because the main thrust is to create conditions that are not conducive to the onset of osteoporosis. In contrast, in secondary prevention the aim is to eliminate predisposing risk factors that, if allowed to progress, would accelerate the development of osteoporosis. Such risk factors may be conditions that are associated with osteoporosis (such as hyperthyroidism or Cushing's syndrome) or they may be the first indications of the onset of the disease (such as fracture of the proximal femur or vertebral crush fracture), which require treatment in order to prevent further damage.[1]

General health

The old adage 'prevention is better than cure' is as true today as when it was first used, especially in the treatment of osteoporosis. Although there is a genetic predisposition, producing risk factors that are not

RISK FACTOR FOCUS

List of risk factors for osteoporosis	
Modifiable risks	*Non-modifiable risks*
Inactivity	White race
Low calcium in diet	Female gender
Cigarette smoking	Family history
Excessive consumption of protein	Light skin
Caffeine	Small frame
Alcohol	Scoliosis
Vitamin D deficiency	Previous osteoporotic fracture
Low weight for height	Previous bone loss through immobilisation, hyperparathyroidism, thyrotoxicosis, liver disease, malabsorption, rheumatoid arthritis, chronic illness, corticosteroids or phenytoin
Oestrogen deficiency	

under the control of the individual, such as those associated with race, gender and frame type, there are other risk factors, such as cigarette smoking, alcohol consumption and vitamin D deficiency, that can be influenced by preventative measures. In the Risk Factor Focus above, known risks are divided into two main categories depending on whether or not they can be averted.

It can be seen that there are a number of predisposing factors that can result in the development of osteoporosis if not corrected before an individual reaches adulthood. Clearly, the earlier the assessment and proposed intervention, the greater the benefit to the patient.

For prevention to be effective in such a situation, two distinct strategies should be put into practice:

1. A population-based health promotion style programme that highlights the risks of developing the disease and the effects osteoporosis can have in later life. Once interest has been aroused, the emphasis can then be shifted to stress the simple measures that can be instituted to ensure that children grow up aware of these and the benefits to be obtained from following a healthy lifestyle.

2. An individualised programme whereby certain sections of the population known to be at greater risk of a low bone mass density (BMD) are targeted. These would be patients with diseases or undergoing treatments that reduce BMD, or individuals at risk of falling.[2,3]

In an ideal world, these two strategies would be employed in tandem to make sure that resources are aimed at those who need them most. In reality, if there is a lack of political will to carry out these programmes, then progression is dependent on activists or pioneers with a motivational interest. Knowledge of this fact has led informed opinion to bias their guidelines in favour of prevention directed at a case-finding strategy rather than at a global programme.[2,3]

Even armed with this knowledge, there can be obstacles to progress, as the tendency is to hark back to the information gained from the available outmoded data on osteoporosis. The existing information must be analysed and developed into a practical solution, which, while alerting the public at large to a general awareness of osteoporosis and its consequences, can identify and single out those in greatest need of a more tailored programme in order to provide the individual with the greatest benefit.

There are a great many preventative treatments available that could be offered more widely, but these would require to be generally acceptable to people *en masse* or at least to that particular group selected for the treatment. For example, an argument could be made for administering hormone replacement therapy (HRT) to all postmenopausal women because this would prevent the bone loss associated with the menopause. However, such wholesale prescribing would be unacceptable for many reasons, both ethical and financial. Apart from which, it is known from present studies that long-term compliance with HRT extending over a number of years is difficult because of the perceived lack of benefits.

For a widespread HRT strategy to succeed, support for such a scheme would require a detailed educational programme, strict supervision of patients and feedback on the success – or lack of it – of the therapy. It would be the prerogative of the state to decide how such a scheme should be funded, as this type of programme would put an extra burden on the standard medical and pharmaceutical services and would add to the caseload of individual specialist practitioners. As both contraindications and side-effects to HRT exist, such a broad-brush approach would require both precise monitoring to detect adverse effects and prevent complications, and strict management so as to aid compliance.[4]

There are other measures that can be more easily undertaken than the mass prescription of HRT. It is possible, for example, to ensure that everyone in a population has an adequate dietary intake of calcium. Action on this front is already in place in many countries by the addition of calcium to refined flour used in the manufacture of white bread. Such a step enables families on even a limited budget to obtain a calcium supplement in their diet. Extra calcium that is not required by the body is not absorbed, so there is no danger of side-effects by the use of this additive. Bakers in the UK are obliged by law to add calcium to white flour after refining, to ensure that the calcium content is the same as that of wholemeal flour, which has not undergone the refining process. This is a cheap and harmless way in which the Government can provide people, especially children, with extra calcium in the diet.

Another valuable source of calcium is the drinking water. If this is sourced from rainwater that has washed down from limestone hills, leading to calcium being leached from the limestone into the drinking water, it will contain enough calcium to help prevent osteoporosis. But in areas where the water is collected from non-limestone hills or from peaty moorland then the resident population will have a low calcium level in their drinking water and consequently a high incidence of osteoporosis. The regional trend of osteoporosis linked to the calcium content of drinking water may be skewed by the increased use of bottled water, which can have either a low or high content of calcium depending on the source.[5]

Although the addition of fluoride to the water supply remains controversial, it cannot be denied that improvements in the dental health of children have been apparent for a number of years. The evidence of efficacy in the prevention of osteoporosis is less well proven. Studies have shown that some patients in highly fluoridated water areas have shown an increase in bone mass, but there is little evidence of reduction in fractures, probably related to the fact that fluoride has no proven efficacy in this aspect.[6]

Encouraging the population to participate more in active sport and to take more physical exercise has proved beneficial in the long term in the prevention of osteoporosis. It is important to foster these habits in children from an early age in the hope that such activities, participated in throughout the school years, will be carried on into later life. It is therefore imperative that good sport facilities for both children and adults are available in the communities in which they live. Sadly, in recent years such amenities have been seen as a luxury and not every school possesses adequate playing fields, while gymnasiums for adults are often within private members clubs, mainly for the affluent.

Genetic factors

There are a number of both direct and indirect genetic factors that can affect an individual's predisposition to osteoporosis. The direct genetic effects include the inherited gender, ethnic origin, skin type, body frame size and family history. If high risk is identified according to several of these factors, then there is a high risk of osteoporosis. Because these factors are often interlinked it is difficult to isolate one single most important item, as one can be often be a predictor of another.

The indirect genetic factors relate either to conditions that indirectly reduce bone mass, such as thyroid and parathyroid function, or to a course of treatment, usually for a chronic disorder, that affects bone metabolism. The importance of these secondary risks will depend on the severity of the disorder or on the length of time over which treatment has been given.[2]

Fetal development

In the initial stages of development from an embryo into a fetus, prior to birth, the fetus is completely dependent on the mother for nutrition. If the mother's diet is deficient in any way, then this will be transmitted to the developing fetus. During the pregnancy, therefore, it is crucial that there is an ample supply of nutrients to feed the growing fetus at every stage of development. Vitally important is the supply of calcium, which is required for the production of bone throughout the whole period of fetal growth. The greatest demand for calcium is towards the end of pregnancy as the calcium content of the infant reaches 9.6 g/kg just prior to birth; this compares with only 2.1 g/kg at the end of the first trimester. It is good practice to advise mothers to increase their calcium intake in the latter stages of the pregnancy in order to provide sufficient calcium. In the event of the mother not having enough calcium within her blood to supply her developing infant, then there will be some calcium loss from the mother's bone. This loss, however, will not compensate fully for a low dietary intake of calcium and the infant will almost certainly be born with a calcium deficiency and the possibility of bone deformities.[7]

Growing phase

In order to ensure that babies in the early years of life develop to their full potential, all the essential nutrients must be present in their diet. If breastfed, this is not a problem, as the infant is provided for by the mother's milk, which contains plenty of calcium along with the other necessary vitamins and minerals. When the infant is weaned, the products used are generally derived from cow's milk, which again is a rich source of calcium.

For the majority of the population this source of calcium poses no problems, however there are a number of children who are intolerant of cow's milk, because of inherited digestive problems. These children should be given alternative soya-based products, which contain similar nutrients and are fortified to ensure that they provide sufficient vitamins and minerals. Certain ethnic and racial populations are more widely affected by cow's milk intolerance than others. In white European and North American populations only about 5–10% are affected, while in Afro-Caribbean and Asian populations the rate can be as high as 90%.

If a child has an inherited lactase deficiency and cannot tolerate milk products, the main sources of calcium will become bread, vegetables and drinking water. Calcium supplementation will almost always be required, as it is difficult to obtain enough calcium from such a limited diet.[8]

As explained earlier, milk and milk products are the prime dietary sources of calcium for children, particularly during the growing years. In the UK milk used to be provided free to all schoolchildren, thus giving them essential nutrients as part of their daily diet; this government policy was discontinued a number of years ago and has been followed by a general reduction in milk consumption.

With the decline in the drinking of milk as a daily routine, the chief source of calcium in the diet has changed to bread made from calcium-fortified flour. If it were not for this supplementation of bread flour with calcium, then a large percentage of teenagers in the lower social classes in the UK would be calcium deficient. This would be a critical situation for adolescents between the ages of 11 and 15, when the demand for calcium is at its highest; there is also speculation as to whether the recommended daily amount (RDA) of calcium should be raised to 20 mmol in line with the American standard, rather than the British standard of 12.5 mmol. The supplementation of bread flour prevents osteoporosis, not only benefiting the young in ensuring that they have sufficient calcium for growth, but also helping the elderly, especially women, who require more calcium because of their inability to efficiently conserve calcium.[1]

Exercise throughout a child's development is crucial in encouraging bone growth, especially if weight-bearing, as this will lead to increases in bone mass from the constant stresses and strains put upon the bone. Regular exercise should be part of every youngster's everyday activity; this is not always possible with the demands of the school curriculum and other activities, which can be a powerful discouragement for young girls, who would benefit most from attaining the maximum potential peak bone mass. Children sometimes become overweight because they do not actively participate in exercise programmes. This leads to a vicious circle in which overweight children fail to undertake adequate exercise because of their excess weight. However, this is partially compensated for by their bone having to support this extra burden, which results in an increase bone mass in comparison with children of a similar age who are nearer to ideal body weight.

In order to maintain bone mass through the final phase of growth and into adulthood it is important that the all the factors that enable the growth of bone are continued. These factors include regular exercise, plenty of calcium in the diet and enough exposure to sunlight to manufacture vitamin D, which is essential for calcium absorption. Even in late teenage, bone mass can still be gained by optimising these elements. Once the peak bone mass has been attained it is necessary to prevent gradual bone loss by following a diet that is naturally high in calcium, as this will stabilise the bone mass before any appreciable bone loss can take place. A diet containing a high calcium content is necessary for pregnant women, since the developing fetus will draw calcium from the mother's bone if there is insufficient in the diet. The level of calcium must also be maintained at a high level throughout breastfeeding, as lactation requires extra calcium in the diet. Women who have not had sufficient calcium during pregnancy and lactation may well develop osteoporosis in later life.

To protect herself from a premature loss of bone mass while menstruating, it is important for a woman to maintain a high level of oestrogen, which creates the environment for protecting bone mass. A woman who enters the menarche early and becomes postmenopausal late in life will have a higher bone mass and maintain that mass for a longer time than someone who starts menstruating late in life and finishes early. If levels of oestrogen are supplemented by the use of an oral contraceptive, this may also have an effect on increasing bone mass.[9]

Adulthood

There is a common misconception that once adulthood is reached, there is nothing more that an individual can do to prevent the slow descent into middle age and the progress into old age. This is far from the truth, as there are a number of factors within adult life that can be managed or eliminated to obtain and maintain a good quality of life, well into old age. This has already been proved in the case of heart disease, in which efforts to promote healthy living have been shown to have made a huge difference in prevention; the same approach can be applied to osteoporosis, and it has been proved that good habits will indeed delay the onset of the disease. The main areas of interest are lifestyle, diet and, for women, the menopause. These points are discussed below.

Lifestyle factors

Various habits can affect bone mass and thus increase or reduce the risk of osteoporosis. These are discussed more fully in the following chapter, but in summary, the three main areas are alcohol consumption, physical exercise and cigarette smoking. All these activities have an effect on the formation of bone, bone turnover and maintaining bone strength. Therefore they require to be discussed with individuals, no matter whether the advice is being given on (a) the prevention of long-term bone loss, or (b) the reduction of further bone loss in severe disease.

The earlier these subjects are discussed the better, as often, once bad habits develop the effort required to make a change is considerable; particularly when the habit is seen as a pleasure, indulged in as one of the luxuries of life.

Diet

A balanced nutritional diet is important in the prevention of osteo-porosis. The essential constituents are calcium, vitamins, especially D, energy and a moderate, but not excessive, amount of protein.

It is difficult to relate the onset of osteoporosis to a low calcium intake in adulthood, as the bone mass is more dependent on the calcium intake in childhood and thus the current calcium intake may not be particularly relevant. Furthermore, the ability of the body to absorb calcium decreases with age due to parathyroid hormone increase; this secondary hyperparathyroidism increases bone turnover, leading to bone loss. Therefore it is necessary to ensure the correct calcium intake at each stage of life in order to maintain bone metabolism (see Management Focus, below).

Vitamin D deficiency is known to cause abnormal bone formation, as is seen in the childhood disease called rickets, which occurs in communities where vitamin D intake is low in the diet or subcutaneous

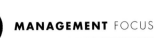

MANAGEMENT FOCUS

Total daily calcium requirements at all ages of life[16]	
Age group	*Daily calcium (mg)*
Infants from birth to 1 year	400–600
Children	
1–5 years	800
6–10 years	800–1200
Adolescents/young adults 11–24 years	1200–1500
Men	
25–65 years	1000
Over 65 years	1500
Women	
25–50 years	1000
Pregnant and lactating	1200
Postmenopausal on oestrogens	1000
Postmenopausal but not on oestrogens	1500
Over 65 years	1500

production is limited because of low levels of exposure to sunlight. Vitamin D has also been reported to be necessary for muscle condition and its absence will increase body sway and hence lead to a tendency to fall. The body's ability to both store and manufacture the active moieties of vitamin D diminishes with age; this has led to a recommendation that daily intakes be increased from the normal adult daily dose of 200 IU to 400 IU for those between 50 and 70 years of age and 800 IU for those over 70 years.

A diet high in protein and phosphate (in excess of 1 g protein per kg per day) may lead to high levels of urea and calcium in the urine (hypercalciuria). If this is not corrected by altering the diet, the body will try to compensate by releasing increased levels of parathyroid hormone. This secondary hyperparathyroidism will cause qualitative micro-architectural abnormalities in the bone. A high intake of fibre containing various chelating agents, including phytic and oxalic acids, may reduce the absorption of calcium from the intestine because of the formation of insoluble chelates of calcium.[10]

Malnutrition, whether it is unintentional as a result of a lack of self-care in an elderly person, or self-inflicted as a result of anorexia and bulimia, is likely to lead to a reduction in bone mass. In menstruating women a reduction in weight below a critical level will also lead the cessation of menstruation (amenorrhoea), which causes a decrease in the secretion of oestrogen. The lack of oestrogen leads to a loss of the protective effect on bone mass conservation; even just a few months of amenorrhoea will cause a significant loss of bone mass, which may never be fully regained before the onset of the menopause.

Menopause

Although peak bone mass is lower in women than in men, once this peak is attained the rate of decline is roughly at the same rate in the two sexes, about 0.25% to 1% per year. In women, this decline continues until the approach of the menopause, when the bone loss becomes dramatic during the next five years. Postmenopausally, the rate of bone loss once again matches that of men.

The critical period is the three years just prior to the menopause, when a woman will start to experience bouts of amenorrhoea, which can last for one or two cycles at a time. This amenorrhoea is the precursor to a dramatic loss of bone mass and can be predicted from a decline in the levels of circulating sex hormones oestrogen and progesterone. After the menopause, the body homeostasis is realigned and the rate of bone loss reduces to a level that is closer to that prior to the menopause and similar to that of men of the same age.

Bone loss during the menopause is a result of lowered oestrogen levels, leading to an increase of bone resorption by up to 85% and a compensating increase in bone formation by up to 45%. The rates at which bone loss occurs appears to vary from person to person within a population, creating a normal distribution of fast and slow bone losers. The difference can be as much as 50% over a 12-year period, calculated using the biochemical markers serum total alkaline phophatase, urinary calcium and hydroxyproline. Therefore, not every woman going through the menopause will suffer sufficient bone loss to require either preventative therapy or treatment.[3]

Secondary osteoporosis

It is important to prevent secondary causes of osteoporosis. There are several conditions that can lead to osteoporosis, if not kept under control. Amongst these are diseases of the parathyroid and thyroid function; such malfunctions lead to reduced calcium intake, creating a lack of the calcium that is necessary for bone maintenance. Similarly, there are a few inflammatory and gastrointestinal diseases that prevent the normal intake and regulation of the necessary nutrients for bone production, leading to a net bone mass loss.

Various inherited conditions of bone and the kidneys, such as osteogenesis imperfecta and homocystinuria, will produce osteoporosis. These conditions must be diagnosed in the early stages, in order that treatment can be given to limit the long-term effects of the disease on mobility and quality of life.

Some drugs can also induce osteoporosis, especially when used in long-term therapy for the maintenance of remission in a chronic disease. This effect should be taken into consideration at the start of any course of treatment. If necessary, preventative osteoporosis therapy should be given in conjunction with the active treatment for the chronic disease, otherwise the patient may have their primary condition controlled but develop osteoporosis as a result of the treatment. The drugs to be aware of in this context are the corticosteroids, heparin and the antiepileptics, which all cause changes to the bone by altering the availability of the required nutrients.

Men

Although men do not undergo a phase equivalent to the menopause and the ensuing associated rapid loss of bone mass, they are not exempt from osteoporosis and may still derive some good from preventive treatment measures. Men benefit not only from the absence of a menopause but also from a higher normal peak bone mass and are therefore at much less risk of developing osteoporosis in later life. However, the longer a man lives, the greater his chances of developing osteoporosis; this is more likely in the present day, because life expectancy in industrialised countries is so much longer than it used to be, beyond the traditional three score years and ten. To counteract this, men should ensure that they avoid overindulgence in food that is rich in protein, and should follow a routine that includes plenty of weight-bearing exercise, in order to prevent the natural bone loss that comes with age.[10]

The high incidence of fracture seen in women with osteoporosis during and after the menopausal years does not occur to the same extent in men of a similar age. However, if all the known differences are taken into account, including the presence of risk factors, the pathology of osteoporosis in both men and women is the same. Taking all the foregoing circumstances into account, once men have reached the same absolute bone mineral density as women, by which time men are usually much older, the fracture risk is equal. It follows then that men should be given full information on all the aspects of osteoporosis, its development and the measures to be taken to prevent it and the therapies that can benefit them.[3]

Fractures

If a great deal of bone loss has occurred and the patient is diagnosed as having osteoporosis, the current treatments available may be able to reverse some of the detrimental effects of the disease. The most significant complication of osteoporosis is the occurrence of a related fracture, which can restrict activity, mobility and, in severe cases, result in a fatality. Thus, it is essential to reduce the risk of a fracture to prevent the downward spiral of events leading to morbidity and mortality. Osteoporotic fractures are more often than not associated with a fall; if this is in a frail and elderly patient the likelihood of related complications is high. Hence, it is imperative that if a frail elderly person has either a diagnosis of osteoporosis or is thought to be developing osteoporosis then the potential risk of a fall should be considered. Every effort should be made to reduce the risk of such an occurrence, in an attempt to prevent a fracture.

There are two main methods of preventing fractures: the first is to ensure that the bone is as strong as possible, by giving treatment for the prevention of the further loss of bone mass. These are all factors that have been discussed before, such as a good diet with sufficient calcium, vitamin D and other essential nutrients; lifestyle factors – low alcohol intake, plenty of exercise and cessation of smoking. The second method of preventing falls and injuries is to look at the individual and isolate all those parameters that could contribute to a fall (see Risk Factor Focus, below), then eliminate or reduce the risk if at all possible.

The elderly are at greater risk of a fall because their muscle power is weaker due to loss of flexibility and the poor coordination that occurs with age. This is why older people are more prone than younger people to slip, trip or stumble and eventually fall. If the fall is particularly traumatic and involves injury, then the older person may be too weak and frail to get up. This can lead to secondary complications if the person remains on the floor for any length of time. The direction of the fall can also be critical: a fall to the side rather than to the front increases the likelihood of a hip fracture. Of those elderly people who fall, one in five will require medical attention and one in 40 will be hospitalised. If osteoporosis is present then a fracture may occur; 25% of those sustaining a fracture will die and 50% will not be able to live independently again.

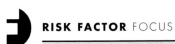

Identifiable risk factors for falls
Muscle weakness
Abnormality of gait or balance
Poor eyesight
Drug therapy – hypnotics, sedatives, diuretics, antihypertensives
Neurological disease, e.g. Parkinson's disease, stroke
Foot problems/arthritis
Layout of home environment (e.g. loose or slippery floor covering)

It is known that between 2.5 and 12% of people aged 65 or over will suffer a fracture sustained after a fall while living in the community. Having fallen once, an elderly person will be afraid of falling again and will tend to restrict their activity. The effect of this is that they become more dependent on others, leading to social isolation and a deterioration in their physical and mental ability to cope with life on their own.

A number of clinical studies have examined various strategies and interventions to help reduce the number of falls sustained by elderly persons living either in the community or in institutions, such as care homes or hospitals. These studies have proved that it is possible to reduce the incidence of falls by between 20 and 50% by introducing exercises designed to improve balance and muscle strength. These enable a person to walk with a more balanced stride, improving the ability to cope with uneven surfaces. In one study, a group of people over the age of 80 and at risk of falling were divided into two groups; the control group received normal care, while the others followed a programme consisting of a number of repetitive exercises, including some ankle-strengthening movements. These exercises were performed regularly in the patient's own home, over a six-month period. At the same time, the members of the exercise group were encouraged to take regular exercise for a 30-minute period, three times a week. This programme was undertaken for a year. At the end of this time, the findings showed that there was a 30% reduction in falls by those who had participated in the exercise programme compared with those patients in the control group. Where possible, environmental hazards were either removed or reduced to a minimum in both groups, so that the participants could cope better with the activities of daily life. Any medication that could cause loss of balance was either changed or withdrawn to eliminate this factor.[11]

The use of hip protectors has been studied in a few clinical trials. These are either of plastic or of foam padding and fit into pockets in specially designed underwear. If an elderly patient is liable to fall no matter what means are employed to prevent the fall, the theory is that the wearing of such protection will prevent injury following a fall. Hip protectors have had a modicum of success, showing a reduction in hip fractures; but unfortunately this was not statistically significant.[12] This lack of effectiveness, coupled with the bulky and uncomfortable nature of the product, makes them unacceptable to the majority of elderly people. Hip protectors are available on the National Health Service but are not routinely stocked because of the low demand.

A major contributing factor to the probability of a fracture, particularly of the vertebrae, is the presence of a primary factor. In a study of postmenopausal women, subjects were divided into those who had a vertebral fracture at the beginning of the study and those who had not. After a one-year period, the groups were examined to establish the existence of any subsequent fractures. This study was an analysis of three large osteoporosis trials carried out on women who were over 20 years postmenopausal. The research discovered that if a woman had had a vertebral fracture prior to the commencement of the trial she was fivefold more likely to suffer a further fracture within the following year compared with a woman who had no previous history of vertebral fracture. The analysis of the data suggests that after reaching the point of a primary fracture, osteoporosis quickly progresses to a stage at which other fractures will occur.[13]

The use of certain drugs in the elderly is known to increase the possibility of falls, and hence subsequent bone fractures. These include drugs that cause central nervous system depression, leading to sedation and an alteration in the ability to coordinate voluntary muscle activity. For example, the psychotropic drugs, including the older tricyclic antidepressants, the selective serotonin reuptake inhibitors, sedatives, especially the longer acting benzodiazepines, and antipsychotic agents, such as the major tranquillisers may have such effects. Other drugs that may affect balance and hence induce a fall are the antihypertensives, which can cause postural hypotension leading to unsteadiness when standing up normally or when getting up quickly from sitting or lying down. A clinical study examined the possibility that benzodiazepines might not only induce a fall but also be instrumental in causing hip fractures. This study reviewed patients over the age of 65 who had suffered a hip fracture unrelated to a road accident or cancer. It was found that, with the one exception of lorazepam, there was no appreciable link between benzodiazepine use and the incidence of hip fracture. The results also suggested that, although benzodiazepines can increase the rate of falls, they may also help to relax the muscles, reducing the impact of the fall.[14,15]

Self-help groups

In recent years, the increase in the number of people diagnosed with osteoporosis has encouraged the development of self-help groups, consisting of lay and medical people. In the UK, this has led to the development of the National Osteoporosis Society (NOS), which, through a network of local branches and a national centre, helps to fund research and raises awareness by distributing up-to-date information and knowledge of the subject.

These groups tend to appeal primarily to people suffering from the condition, and then to people who have a relative or friend with the disease and wish to be aware of ways in which they can help. Gradually information is distributed to the general public and even promotes the imparting of knowledge to the medical profession on the availability of new products.

These groups have an important role to play in public education, encouraging people to adopt a healthier lifestyle and diet. This has been evident in the increase of requests for calcium carbonate from community pharmacies for the purpose of self-medication. There is a plethora of information available to women who are entering the menopause on the range of treatments possible and advice on which one would best suit them. There is now no need to suffer in silence, as there is help and treatment to prevent symptoms and to improve health throughout their later life.

References

1. Woolf A D, Dixon A S. *Osteoporosis: a Clinical Guide*. London: Martin Dunitz, 1988.
2. Royal College of Physicians. *Osteoporosis. Clinical Guidelines for Prevention and Treatment*. London: Royal College of Physicians, 1999.
3. South African Medical Association – Osteoporosis Working Group. Osteoporosis clinical guideline. *S Afr Med J* 2000; **90**: 907–944.
4. Prevention and treatment of osteoporosis. *MeReC Bull* 1999; **10**(7): 25–28.

5. Matkovic V, Kostial K, Simonovic I, *et al.* Bone status and fracture rates in two regions in Yugoslavia. *Am J Clin Nutr* 1979; **32**: 540–549.

6. Simonen O, Laittinen O. Does fluoridation of drinking water prevent bone fragility in osteoporosis? *Lancet* 1985; **2**: 432–433.

7. *Geigy Scientific Tables.* Basle: Geigy Pharmaceutical Publications, 1970.

8. McNeish A S, Sweet E M, Lactose intolerance in childhood coeliac disease. *Arch Dis Child* 1968; **43**: 433–437.

9. Recker R R, Davies M, Hinders M, *et al.* Bone gain in young adults. *JAMA* 1992; **268**: 2403–2408.

10. Parfitt A M. Dietary risk factors for age related bone loss and fractures. *Lancet* 1983; **2**: 1181–1185.

11. Campbell A J, Robertson M C, Gardener M M, *et al.* Falls prevention over 2 years: a randomised control trial in women 80 years and older. *Age Ageing* 1999; **28**: 513–518.

12. Parker M J. Hip protectors for preventing hip fractures in the elderly people. In: *The Cochrane Library*, Issue 4. Oxford: Update Software, 2002.

13. Wasnich R D, Davis J W, Ross P D. Spine fracture risk is predicted by non-spine fractures. *Osteoporosis Int* 1994; **4**: 1–5.

14. Pierfitte C, Macouillard G, Thicoïpe M, *et al.* Benzodiazepines and hip fractures in elderly people: case-control study. *BMJ* 2001; **322**: 704–708.

15. NHS Centre for Reviews and Dissemination. Preventing falls and subsequent injury in older people. *Effective Health Care Bull* 1996; **2**(4): 1–16.

16. NIH Consensus Statement. *Optimal Calcium Intake.* Bethesda, MD: National Institutes of Health, June 1994.

4

Lifestyle factors

The effects of osteoporosis can have a seriously restrictive influence on a person's lifestyle; this is an important consideration in the outcome of the disorder. In most cases, it is not until the patient sustains a fracture that the presence of disease is detected. Therefore, it is at this point that time should be set aside to explain the specific implications of certain lifestyles.

The increase in the incidence of osteoporosis can be attributed to a number of practices – smoking, alcohol abuse and lack of exercise – that are currently prevalent in Western society and that may both prevent adults achieving their optimum bone mass and lead to an increased propensity to loss of bone mass throughout life. This creates a situation in which the development of osteoporosis throughout the ageing population is more certain than not: a third of women and one in 12 men over 50 years will suffer an osteoporotic fracture at some time in their life. How their quality of life is affected will depend on the type of fracture sustained, although the outcome will usually be a reduction in both independence and mobility.

Hip fractures almost always cause loss of mobility and independence and in extreme cases can be the root cause of death. The more common vertebral fractures will have a slower incremental effect on spine curvature, leading to loss of height and the compression of internal organs, breathlessness from the lungs and oesophageal reflux from the gastrointestinal tract. These effects and the associated restrictions on normal daily life activities can induce mental health problems, such as depression.

The importance of health promotion and the need to inform the general public of these facts, making them aware of these problems created in later life by this disease, is one reason why the National Osteoporosis Society (NOS) has produced literature for a number of health groups aimed at developing a prevention strategy. The literature was designed to be used in public and health-related venues to alert members of the public to the risks they may be running of developing osteoporosis. As a part of this programme, health professionals, both practitioners and those involved in making decisions on health strategies, were informed of those patients who were at greatest risk of succumbing to osteoporosis. The aim was to target those patients requiring further investigation and those in need of advice on the measures they should take in order to prevent the onset of the disease. The NOS also supplied guidelines on how to inform the general public, carry out surveys into the prevalence of osteoporosis amongst the population, and how to go about obtaining the necessary resources for such a task.[1]

This type of measure is known as primary prevention, because it aims to direct general information – in this case on lifestyle – to as many people as possible in order to bring about small changes in behaviour. For this type of project to be successful, it is essential that the information messages are distributed via the popular media, that is television, radio and print. This must be enforced by more detailed information, giving the answers to all the common questions through the formal health promotion mechanism. The messages should be clear and concise, and delivered in a manner that will motivate people to make that change. Unfortunately it is always more difficult to convince younger people, who would be the greatest beneficiaries of such knowledge, since the major benefits will be manifested in the longer term and lie too far into the future to be given much consideration at present. In this instance, it may prove more productive to emulate the techniques commonly used in the marketing industry, such as peer group pressure, celebrity endorsement or sex appeal rather than the more usual health promotional methods.

In order to be a success, a prevention programme cannot rely solely on a promotional campaign through the media, it needs to be supported by a parallel programme aimed at health professionals, making sure that they are spelling out the same message. These health professionals will normally operate on a one-to-one basis with their patients, encouraging them to improve their lifestyle and, in so doing, to exert an influence also on the people with whom the patient comes in contact.

In any group there will always be individuals who are more motivated than others to adopt new practices and to respond to new challenges; these people can be persuaded to influence their peers to do likewise. Vitally important amongst these groups are mothers to be, mothers of young children and the elderly. Mothers are, in the main, the ones who decide the family's diet; how the children are brought up and generally set the pattern of the family's lifestyle and have the ability to win over the reluctant father. Elderly people can be motivated by the prospect of maintaining as active a lifestyle as possible and will

LIFESTYLE FACTOR FOCUS

Lifestyle factors to consider in the prevention of osteoporosis
Alcohol
Smoking
Diet
Exercise

generally prove amenable to gentle changes, which will work to their own advantage.

The health promotional material should not be restricted to normal venues such as the doctor's surgery or the local community pharmacist, but placed in a wide variety of locations in order to reach all sections of the community, such as schools, shops, offices, workplaces, leisure centres and libraries. Similarly, health visitors, social service workers and the catering staff of large organisations should also be enlisted in the campaign. This will ensure that the people at greatest risk and those who must adopt a healthier lifestyle cannot fail to be aware of the disease prevention information.

The people at greatest risk will more than likely be already attending one of the various branches of the health service, for example the primary care team, accident and emergency department or a specialist clinic such as gynaecology, rheumatology or orthopaedics. These high-risk individuals should be adequately catered for by the available health services, although, sadly, for these patients it is often too late to arrest the onset of the disease, as the osteoporosis is well developed and medication is required to halt the progress of the disease. Those people at medium to low risk are the ones who will derive the greatest benefits from being given the correct information and re-education on how to follow a healthy lifestyle in order to prolong and maintain their health.[2]

The information in health promotion on the prevention of osteoporosis is concerned with the factors listed in the Lifestyle Factor Focus above.

The prevalence, or absence, of these lifestyle factors can be ingrained from a young age, as often children will follow on a pattern set by their parents. It is important, therefore, to ensure that advantages of adopting good habits and not bad ones are understood from an early age.[3,4]

Alcohol

Because of the influence of alcohol on behaviour, particularly where the young are concerned, it has posed an increasing problem in Western society. In recent years, this problem has been exacerbated by the ready availability and variety of forms in which such drinks are marketed. Some forms of alcohol have been sweetened and made to look and taste like soft drinks, so that it is often difficult to distinguish between alcoholic and non-alcoholic beverages. The two major consequences of the appearance of these sweetened alcoholic drinks on the market have been to encourage consumption of alcohol at an ever earlier age and to create a fashion in experimentation with these drinks, often to excess. In particular, alcohol consumption by young women has risen alarmingly in recent years.

Overindulgence in alcohol has been shown to be detrimental to the development of peak bone mass in young men and women. This is more disadvantageous to women, because their peak bone mass is generally lower than that of men and because of the effect of the menopause in lowering bone mass in later life. In certain areas in which alcohol consumption is high, this can be the most important lifestyle risk factor for osteoporosis.

Alcohol is known to be poisonous to bone, causing a decrease in serum osteocalcin, osteoblast proliferation and activity. Overall, this has a direct effect on bone strength, manifesting as a change in bone histology and as a reduction in bone formation. Alcohol has been shown to modify the action of the skeletal signalling peptides, causing them to alter their response to bone cells and to these regulatory peptides. This further affects the activity of bone cells, increasing bone resorption by osteoclasts and reducing the bone-forming osteoblast activity.

In an individual who has consumed a high level of alcohol over a lengthy period of time, for instance as witnessed in chronic alcoholism, nutrition is affected. One of the consequences of this is a lower intake of vitamins, particularly vitamin D. In severe cases, this malnourished state may be compounded by cirrhosis of the liver together with a pseudo-Cushing's syndrome. Other indirect effects of alcohol on bone include the imbalance in the actions of calcium-regulating hormones, mineral homeostasis and bone loading through a reduction in body weight. Further disturbances of nutrition can lead to hypomagnesaemia and hypocalcaemia, which will further reduce the individual's ability to maintain bone mass. If a degree of liver failure develops, then vitamin D metabolism will be affected, leading to reduced absorption, a shortened active biological half-life and sometimes reduced levels of the hydroxy metabolites of vitamin D. Reduced levels of 1,25-dihydroxy-vitamin D can either directly affect bone metabolism or can indirectly affect the body's regulation of calcium by causing a malfunction of the parathyroid hormone, leading to a condition of hypocalcaemia. Although some effects on calcium regulation are seen with these disturbances of calcium-regulating hormones, it is the overall effect on mineral homeostasis that creates the problems of bone mass maintenance.

Chronic alcoholics will, in the majority of cases, have a low BMD, although this may not be exclusively due to the direct and indirect effects of alcohol on bone formation. Two factors contribute to the effect of alcohol on the skeleton: one is the peak blood alcohol level and the other the duration of the alcohol consumption. It has been shown that excessive alcohol intake decreases bone remodelling and creates a negative remodelling balance, but it is not possible to predict how much alcohol will have this effect. In men, this decrease in bone remodelling has the effect of doubling the risk of fracture neck of femur. In women there is a contradictory response depending on whether it is before or after the menopause: premenopausal alcohol consumption has the expected effect of reducing BMD, but in postmenopausal women an increase in BMD is seen. It is not clear why this should happen, but it is thought to be related to the observation that oestrogen production in adipose tissue is enhanced by alcohol, which stimulates the release of calcitonin, a hormonal inhibitor of bone resorption. It is also thought that the reduction in bone remodelling seen with alcohol consumption helps to reduce bone loss in the postmenopausal woman and the young male. This effect of alcohol on women can help to reduce bone loss caused by the loss of oestrogen while going through the menopause. In contrast, in the young male, although there is reduction in bone remodelling, no visual change is apparent in outward appearance; nevertheless the loss of bone architecture will, in later life, increase fracture risk.

There is known to be a communication link between osteoclasts and osteoblasts, so that they work together to ensure the maintenance of bone mass. This is thought to be achieved via a 'coupling factor', possibly a peptide, produced by osteoblasts and deposited into the mineralised bone matrix as part of the cycle of bone formation. As part of the remodelling process, the osteoclasts release the peptide from the matrix, where it is free to stimulate osteoblasts again. Thus it is thought that alcohol does not have a direct effect on osteoblasts, but on the signalling peptides that influence the activity of osteoblasts and osteoclasts.

Another means by which alcohol may affect bone remodelling is by disturbing the action of cytokines. Two cytokines involved in bone remodelling are known to be affected in this way by alcohol, namely insulin-like growth factor-I and tumour necrosis factor.

Research undertaken on the effect of alcohol on the skeleton is difficult to interpret as the majority of studies have been carried out on alcoholics, who tend to have a complicated medical history. There are many factors that can contribute to the loss of bone mass in conjunction with alcohol consumption, such as nutritional status, magnesium and zinc deficiency, reduced mechanical loading due to lack of exercise and weight loss, malabsorption related to chronic pancreatitis, cigarette smoking and the use of aluminium-containing indigestion remedies. Many individuals often either lie about their consumption of alcohol or, because of the affect of the alcohol, cannot remember how much they have imbibed. One reason, for the wide variation in the results of the studies could be that the age, weight and diet of the individual was not accorded the same degree of importance as the level of alcohol intake. For example, a comparison between a young man of a fairly solid build and an older, lighter man who had been consuming alcohol over a longer period and hence showed a greater bone mass loss, would always show a discrepancy in the skeletal effects of alcohol.

Laboratory experiments in rats have shown that in the short term there is a temporary reduction in calcium levels in the blood after the administration of alcohol. After the chronic administration to growing male rats there was a decrease in bone strength, bone density and the volume of the core of the bone. The result of this, after a ten-month period, was that there was cortical bone loss because of lack of bone formation, and although the vitamin D metabolites were not affected, osteopenia had started to develop. These results in laboratory animals could well reflect the properties of alcohol use in humans, suggesting that young people who start drinking alcohol in large quantities at an early age may suffer as a consequence of effects on their growth pattern.[5]

A comparable picture was seen in experiments on female rats, in which the alcohol-inhibited bone growth led to a failure to achieve expected peak bone mass. Even when the alcohol was discontinued, the female rats did not reach normal bone mass or display the usual mechanical properties; instead osteopenia developed because of the inhibition of bone formation. Again this evidence may reflect the situation in humans; women who have indulged in excessive alcohol consumption in their youth will enter the menopause with a lower than expected bone mass and thus run increasing risk of a fracture at an earlier age than they would have done.

The risk of alcoholism leading to established osteoporosis has been studied only in men, where it has not been thought to be a problem, because complications such as fractures have not materialised. In women, it is believed that alcohol even when taken to excess does not constitute so great a problem, as this is overwhelmed by the effect of the menopause.

Clearly it is difficult to establish if there is an increased risk of osteoporotic fractures in alcoholics. A number of studies have examined this retrospectively, either by analysing the incidence of fractures in alcoholic patients, or by attempting to establish whether patients with fractures showed evidence of alcohol abuse. From these studies, conflicting results were obtained, as fractures were found to be more common in alcoholics than in non-alcoholics in some instances and less frequent in others. In general, it seems that men who abuse alcohol are more likely to be at risk of a fracture, but women are at a reduced risk of a fracture if they drink alcohol to excess. The reason for this may be that when a fracture occurs in an alcoholic, it is associated with trauma rather than the expected osteopenia. Therefore, although the bones may be weakened by the alcohol, the overriding factor is the ability of alcohol to alter balance and precipitate a fall, not the effect on bone.

In conclusion, it is known that alcohol abuse, particularly in men is a risk factor for osteoporosis; animal research modelling the use of alcohol has shown definite changes in bone mass and strength. Endeavouring to find evidence of these bone changes in humans has led to conflicting results concerning bone mass, bone strength, bone architecture and fracture risk. Therefore, as the level of alcohol intake required to produce these changes is unknown; it would be more productive to advise a low or minimum intake of alcohol, since a moderate consumption could be regarded as a risk factor in osteoporosis in men and premenopausal women. Further research is necessary to ascertain the role of alcohol in bone formation and remodelling, and to establish the risk of osteoporosis and fracture. This research should concentrate on finding possible countermeasures, either as a limit to alcohol consumption or as a means of identifying those at greatest risk.[6]

Cigarette smoking

A number of studies have examined the links between cigarette smoking and the incidence of back pain, sciatica and spinal degenerative disease. The findings indicate that back-related problems are more common in smokers and spinal surgery is four times more likely to be practised upon smokers compared with age-matched non-smokers. Surgeons are reputed to have stated that smokers make up 60–70% of the caseload of back procedures.[7]

The relation of back pain to smoking is further illustrated by the finding that the more years a person has smoked the more likely back pain is to be present. This is particularly true for people over the age of 50. It has also been established that there is a connection between smoking and back pain in those who undertake physically demanding work.

Studies of female twins in which comparisons were made between a smoker and a non-smoker by measuring bone mineral density, have shown that prior to the menopause, the smoker displayed a significant reduction of BMD in both the spine and the pelvis.

From this evidence it can be seen that smoking has a significant effect on BMD, and the longer an individual has been smoking the greater the effect, particularly in women. In recent years there has been a trend towards young people smoking at an earlier age, especially in girls. This is manifested by the increasing incidence of lung cancer in women, which has escalated rapidly over the last five years. Smoking at a young age affects the ability of the individual to achieve their potential peak bone mass. Should the smoking continue throughout adult life, then the decline in bone mass will be accelerated, which will be disastrous in women when they enter the menopause and throughout the postmenopausal years.

To what degree the level of smoking affects health – in particular in women – has been questioned. The debate queries whether the effect should be judged over a specific time span, or if the results should be considered over an entire life's consumption. A major advantage to women who have given up smoking will be the beneficial effect of decelerating the rate of bone mass loss.

Smoking does not only reduce bone mass, it also weakens the strength of the bone, which, in turn, leads to an increased risk of hip and vertebral fractures. This premise was confirmed by analysing age-matched patients who had experienced low-impact trauma according to whether they were smokers or non-smokers; it was seen that the potential for fracture was greater in smokers than in non-smokers.

Effects of smoking on bone metabolism

The action of smoking a cigarette produces a cocktail of by-products, ranging from the actual smoke and ash to the tar phase. These

ADVERSE EFFECTS FOCUS

Adverse effects of smoking on bone metabolism

Adverse effect on bone mineral density, accelerated osteoporosis

Impairment of blood flow

Inhibition of osteoblast cellular metabolism

Higher failure rate than expected with spinal fusion

ADVERSE EFFECTS FOCUS

Adverse effects of smoking on sex hormones

Increases metabolism of endogenous and exogenous oestrogen to inactive metabolites

Induces an early menopause and lower body weight

Reduces conversion of peripheral androgens to oestrogens due to a decrease in fat mass

Impairs conversion of peripheral androgens to oestrogens in postmenopausal women

by-products clearly have an impact on bone metabolism, although it is not known exactly how this occurs. There are three main theories: bone degradation, impaired blood flow to the bones and impaired osteoblast metabolism (see Adverse Effects Focus, above).

Accelerated osteoporosis

The combined effects of bone degradation, reduced blood supply and impaired osteoblast function produce an accelerated loss of BMD in people who smoke. In addition, there is also an effect on the sex hormones, particularly oestrogen, which causes an earlier demineralisation of bone; this could also be influenced by nutritional status.

Further dose-dependent effects of smoking on the sex hormones are listed in the Adverse Effects Focus above. These effects could explain why smokers on average experience the menopause earlier than non-smokers and why even when HRT is prescribed to smokers, they do not achieve the same level of hormones as non-smokers.

The slim smoker is often at a disadvantage because of their relatively low oestrogen levels and low bone loading; although the obese smoker has increased bone loading, the benefit of this is countered by the lack of oestrogen. Smoking has affects on other hormones, causing hypercortisolism, hyperthyroidism and calcitonin resistance, all of which have a harmful effect on bone, leading to an increased skeletal bone demineralisation.

The smoker more frequently adopts a lifestyle that includes poor nutrition and a sedentary existence, both predictive of accelerated osteoporosis. Cigarettes produce toxic oxidant free radicals and the likelihood that the smoker's diet is deficient in free radical scavengers, such as vitamin C, vitamin E and beta carotene, leaves them open to greater damage from these toxins.

Impaired blood flow to the bones

Cigarette smoking is well known to cause peripheral vascular disease by reducing the ability of these distant capillaries to perfuse the surrounding tissue. The damage in the peripheral blood vessels is also seen in the blood supply to the spine and the long bones of the skeleton. This consists of vertebral vessel vasoconstriction, endothelial cell, leukocyte and platelet damage, leukocyte and platelet aggregation, leading to changes in the viscosity of blood causing clotting problems and stasis in the smallest of the blood vessels.

The nicotine in cigarette smoke causes damage to the endothelial lining of blood vessels, affecting the release of the vasoconstricting peptide endothelin. The increase in the release of endothelin by cigarette smoking is the major source of a reduced blood flow supply to the periphery and the spine. Nicotine has also been identified as an inhibitor of prostacyclin production, which is responsible for vasodilatation and inhibits platelet aggregation. In the absence of prostacyclin, the blood is unable to flow freely through the vessels and is more liable to clot.

Impaired osteoblast metabolism

A number of the toxic substances produced from cigarette smoking have a detrimental effect on osteoblast activity. These include carbon monoxide, formaldehyde, nitrosamines, benzene, nicotine, benzopyrene and cadmium. It is not completely understood how these affect osteoblasts, but possible theories include damage to mRNA synthesis, impaired deoxyribonucleic acid (DNA) synthesis, inhibition of protein synthesis, inhibition of cellular metabolism and toxic free radical injury. As one of the main toxins in cigarettes, nicotine has been studied extensively and is known to reduce osteoblast cell numbers, prevent collagen synthesis and inhibit osteoblast cellular activity.

Free radicals from cigarette smoke and ash have been found to cause oxidative damage to osteoblast cells, injury to endothelial cells and leukocytes. This is both a short- and long-term effect on the membrane of the involved cells. The osteoblasts also suffer further damage to the mitochondria within the cell, affecting cellular metabolism.

Spinal fusion

In a number of degenerative bone diseases of the spine, it has been shown that if two adjacent vertebrae are fused surgically in order to produce a more rigid spine, this can halt the damage and lessen the symptoms. The chances of this operation being successful are lower in smokers than in non-smokers. This is thought to be because of the more acidic and lower oxygen content of the site in a smoker's body. The two vertebrae that are fused often have a degree of bony demineralisation in smokers, with a poor blood supply and less than the expected number of healthy osteoblasts. This means that the environment in which the fusion is to occur is less than ideal, resulting in a higher failure rate. Delayed non-unions are common, and when a fusion is complete the join is not as strong as that looked for in a similar operation involving a non-smoker. The damage to the surrounding bone also reduces the chance of infiltration of osteoblasts and the accompanying blood supply, which would normally promote healing of the bone graft.[8]

Diet

In order to ensure good bone health throughout life it is important from an early age to eat a good balanced diet, full of the necessary nutrients to enable bone growth to reach its full potential at peak bone mass. A child requires the optimum intake of both calcium and vitamin D from birth, to sustain bone growth and continue to thrive. Improved knowledge of development has shown that pregnant women should increase their calcium intake towards the end of the pregnancy to cater for the demand from the fetus as it prepares for birth. Postnatally, the breast-feeding infant relies on the mother to provide nutrition from breast milk, which is a rich source of the minerals and vitamins necessary for bone growth. The mother must ensure that she has an adequate diet containing sufficient calcium to provide both for herself and for the increased demand made by the infant.

During the growth period, it is important for the child to maintain a diet rich in calcium so that the bone can develop and mature in a healthy manner, without showing any signs of growth problems that were common in children growing up in the cities of Europe in the nineteenth century. Foods that are rich in calcium include dairy products and fortified bread; if a child is unable to eat or has a dislike of any of these products, then reliance is put on fruit and vegetables, which are a poorer source of calcium. Children who do not eat dairy products or bread in large enough quantities to avail themselves of sufficient calcium, should be given supplements.

Vitamin D is the other main ingredient essential to the development of bone. This is derived from the reaction to sunlight of the sterol molecules, which lie just underneath the skin. Usually reserves of vitamin D are built up during the summer months and are drawn upon throughout the winter. If a person fails to gain sufficient exposure to sunlight, a deficiency of vitamin D may result. In order to prevent this, certain standard foods in the UK are fortified with vitamin D, so that everyone can obtain a plentiful supply of this vitamin, despite the low levels of sunlight. Such measures are important in the health of northern Europeans, where the amount and length of sunlight exposure is limited because of the nature of the temperate climate and/or the inability of the sun to penetrate to ground level, particularly in cities where there is an abundance of tall, close-packed buildings.

Although calcium and vitamin D are the main nutrients for good bone health, others, including protein, essential fatty acids, vitamin K, magnesium, phosphorus, potassium and boron are all thought to be important. This would appear to indicate that having a balanced diet with plenty of variety, including fresh fruit and vegetables, which contain all of these nutrients may well protect against bone mass loss.[9,10]

Exercise

Physical exercise can help prevent osteoporosis at all stages of life, but it should be sustained at a reasonably regular level, otherwise the benefits are soon lost. The type of exercise is not as important as the fact that it must be weight-bearing, performed over at least a 40-minute period and undertaken three times a week. Exercise is known to be important in normal bone formation because it is responsible for controlling bone resorption and thus bone loss.

In the early stages of life, up to and including puberty, exercise can help to promote an increase in predicted peak bone mass. In participating children this is reflected in bone density measurements of the hip and lumbar region that are between 2% and 3% greater than those of less active children. Further advantages, such as a change in skeletal geometry and bone turnover may not be reflected by bone biochemical marker measurements. Once peak bone mass has been attained, exercise will reduce the rate of bone loss; this becomes more pronounced in later life. Other benefits of physical exercise include an increase in muscle strength and improved neuromuscular coordination and confidence. Research has yet to define whether there is a specific training exercise programme that will give the maximum benefit in the maintenance or the improvement of bone structure.

The type of exercise undertaken will dictate where in the body the bone mass will be increased, which can lead to a distortion of the overall bone mass. For example, aerobic and weight-bearing exercise increases BMD in the spine, brisk walking can lead to an increased bone density of the hip and aerobic exercise is the only means of increasing the bone mass at the wrist. In order to increase BMD throughout the skeleton it would be best to have a varied exercise programme, using all types of exercises of the body. Furthermore, this varied exercise programme needs to be maintained to ensure that the benefits are continued for as long as possible. A number of studies have shown that, even in post-menopausal women with a depleted BMD, entering an exercise programme can improve bone mass. For example, a group of post-menopausal women who started an exercise programme that included brisk walking, above the anaerobic threshold, for 30 minutes three times a week, showed an increase in BMD in the spine nine months into the programme. The benefit of the exercise was lost, however, if the walking was not so vigorous or the exercise was stopped.[11]

It is worth noting that on its own, exercise only produces a relatively small increase in bone mass, dependent on the intensity of the exercise and frequency of participation. Therefore, although exercise is good at ensuring an adequate peak bone mass in early adulthood, it will not succeed in preventing the significant loss of bone mass that occurs in patients at high risk of fracture.

Excessive exercise can also have a detrimental effect on bone structure, if it is combined with a limited energy and calcium intake from the regular diet. It is then that hypothalamic amenorrhoea or hypogonadism and osteoporosis, with or without fracture, may result. This is most likely to develop in athletes involved in stamina events, such as long-distance running, or in ballet dancers, where fitness and slim profile are important. The level of exercise should be tailored to the individual. Whereas it would be appropriate for a young adult to participate in weight-bearing exercise, for example as in running, this would be ill-advised for an elderly person with known osteoporosis and who is at risk of fracture.[10,12]

Other contributing factors

Although these lifestyle factors can establish the degree of risk of developing osteoporosis and subsequent fracture, there are often other underlying causes. In the prevention of osteoporosis it has been seen that smoking has a direct effect on bone loss, but smoking will also reduce, or even eliminate altogether, the ability to exercise. Similarly, smoking is often combined with alcohol consumption and both contribute to the risk of falling, which may result in a fracture, thus putting the individual at a much greater risk of further damage and leading to an impaired quality of life.

In later life, the simple action of sustaining a fall can have a dramatic effect on the continued quality of life and can induce significant mortality and morbidity. Awareness of this has led to research into the ways by which falls can be prevented and how to reduce the possibility of incurring fracture damage.

 RISK FACTOR FOCUS

Risks associated with likelihood of falling	
Physical factors	*Inducing drugs*
Cognitive dysfunction	Sedatives and hypnotics
Gait	Antidepressants
Balance disorders	Antihypertensives
Weakness	Hypoglycaemic agents
Decreased mobility	Loop diuretics
Visual impairment	
History of falls	

One outcome of this work has been to categorise the risk of falling into (a) physical parameters and (b) those that are drug induced. These are listed in the Risk Factor Focus above.

In the elderly and those with established disease, an analysis should be made of each individual at risk of falling. First, any drug therapy should be assessed in order to establish if this can be discontinued or modified to reduce risk. The most important drugs are the long-acting sedatives, tranquillisers and hypnotics, which constitute the single greatest reversible risk to the elderly. Then ways in which muscle strength and balance could be improved should be investigated. It is possible to design an exercise programme for elderly people at risk that will improve both balance and gait, leading to the strengthening of the weakened muscles. This exercise programme will identify the weakened muscles that have contributed to previous falls or that have encouraged changes in gait and balance.

The home environment can be surveyed to reduce any potential hazards that could be instrumental in leading to a fall. Items to be considered for modification are: slippery surfaces, poor lighting, objects that could be tripped over, for example loose rugs and mats, inappropriate furniture and inadequate footwear. Once this analysis has been completed and the risk of falling lessened as far as possible, if any likelihood of a fall remains then the wearing of padded hip protectors can be considered. In a susceptible individual, these can help reduce the possibility of a fracture from a sideways fall by up to 50%.

References

1. *Osteoporosis – Are You at Risk?* (leaflet). London: National Osteoporosis Society, 2000.
2. Stott P. A time bomb ticks in our bones. *Health and Ageing* January 2001; 30–33.
3. Royal College of Physicians. *Osteoporosis. Clinical Guidelines for Prevention and Treatment*. London: Royal College of Physicians, 1999.
4. Lifestyle advice for fracture prevention. *Drugs Ther Bull* 2002; **40**: 83–86.
5. Peng T C, Cooper C W, Munson P L. The hypocalcaemia of alcohol in rats and dogs. *Endocrinology* 1972; **91**: 586–593.
6. Turner R T. Skeletal response to alcohol. *Alcohol Clin Exp Res* 2000; **24**: 1693–1701.
7. Porter S E, Hanley E N. The musculoskeletal effects of smoking. *J Am Acad Orthop Surg* 2001; **9**: 9–17.
8. Haddley M N, Reddy S V. Smoking and the human vertebral column. *Neurosurgery* 1997; **41**: 116–124.

9.   Department of Health. Nutrition and Bone Health: with particular reference to calcium and vitamin D. Report on Health and Social Subjects 49, 1998.
10. Blair S N, Horton E, Leon A S, *et al.* Physical activity, nutrition and chronic disease. *Med Sci Sports Exerc* 1996; **28**: 335–349.
11. Dalsky G P, Stocke K S, Ehsani A A, *et al.* Weight bearing exercise training and bone mineral content in postmenopausal women. *Ann Intern Med* 1988; **108**: 824–828.
12. Reid I R. Therapy of osteoporosis: calcium, vitamin D and exercise. *Am J Med Sci* 1996 **312**: 278–286.

5

Monitoring the condition

At this stage, there is a need to add depth and detail to the outline given in the preceding chapters. In this chapter there will be more specific information regarding the diagnosis and monitoring of osteoporosis. In particular, recent changes in the diagnosis and differential diagnosis of osteoporosis and the progress made in establishing the causes, together with a certain prognosis, will be elaborated upon. Over the last few decades there have been a number of improvements in diagnostic techniques that have improved the quality and ease of detecting osteoporosis at an early stage, which is where treatment can make a significant difference. Prior to these advances it was difficult to determine the presence of osteoporosis, as the available diagnostic techniques were effective only in identifying the latter stages of the disease by confirming the diagnosis from the symptoms as presented.

Diagnosis

The clinical signs and symptoms of a disease will usually define the predicted outcome based on previous experience, but where osteoporosis is concerned the first indication is often a fracture of the hip, wrist or spine, which could be considered to be an outcome. If this outcome is not investigated further, then the sign could be viewed as a single clinical event, rather than a predictor of a series of episodes, indicative of a specific disease. This may result in osteoporosis being overlooked as a possible diagnosis if at the first presentation the reasons for the fracture are not followed by further diagnostic tests.

Initially, osteoporosis is a condition without apparent symptoms; there are no early warning signs of the underlying damage that exists in the bones, nor of any imminent fractures. It is not until the deterioration of the bones has reached a stage at which the manifestation of a fracture is determined by a low-impact injury that the presence of the disease is suspected. If at this point a diagnosis is not made, then further fractures will result as the degeneration of the bones continues without corrective measures.

The diagnosis of osteoporosis in the early stages of the disease may be deduced from a patient's clinical history and any inherent risk factors. Once an assessment of the probability of osteoporosis has been made, it is then necessary to employ a range of diagnostic tests in order to confirm the degree to which the disease has advanced, the likely prognosis and the possible treatment options to prevent a detrimental outcome.[1]

Body measurements

It is well known that as part of the ageing process there is a slow but discernible loss in height caused by the narrowing of the intervertebral disc and flattening of the vertebrae. This shrinkage for each of the vertebra is small, but overall can amount to around 3 mm loss of height per year. Patient height measurements should be carried out at the same time each day, as there is a variation by as much as 1 cm per day in height throughout the day, depending on the level of hydration of the disc. Hydration is greatest in the morning and lowest at the end of the day, and the best time to measure height is in the afternoon, when the hydration level is relatively stable.

Most people with osteoporosis experience a greater than normal loss in height over time. The degree of loss is dependent on the severity of the osteoporosis; in extreme cases, it can amount to as much as 10 cm in a year. The rate of loss is not linear with time; initially, there is a rapid loss due to an accelerated shrinkage in discs and vertebrae, then the rate is slower, perhaps because shrinkage is limited and perhaps because of stabilisation as the ribs are lowered onto the pelvic bone. Measurement of loss of height is a useful tool to assess patients at risk of osteoporosis and to monitor treatment effectiveness in preventing further height loss.

The method used to measure height may need to be adapted because of difficulty caused by the gradual curvature of the spine due to the effect of osteoporosis. It is sometimes helpful to measure the patient while they are sitting down, measuring only the changes in the lower area of the thoracic spine. Accuracy can be improved by the use of an orthopaedic ruler to mark the spine at a specific point and the use of an X-ray of that section of the spine, taking the measurement from the chair to the marker on the spine.[2]

Radiological techniques

In the main, conventional X-rays of the skeleton are employed to establish the severity and nature of a fracture. These are used to determine

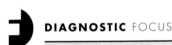

Radiological techniques used in osteoporosis diagnosis

Conventional X-rays
  Back
  Hip
  Finger

Photodensitometry

Photon absorptiometry
  Single-beam
  Dual-beam (DEXA)

Quantitative computed tomography (QCT)

Radioisotopes

---

the interventions required to aid the healing of the injury. However, in the osteoporotic patient, unless extensive X-rays are performed of the spine, proximal hip and other areas, then the root cause of the problem will not be found. Further extensive X-rays are needed not only to detect the presence of fractures, but also to indicate the degree of damage to the bone. For example, a spinal X-ray will allow the practitioner to distinguish the three types of vertebral fracture: crush, wedge or concave. Such fractures of the spine, in particular the crush fracture, are indicative of a more severe form of osteoporosis.

The use of conventional skeletal X-rays in this way to ascertain a low bone mass is unreliable, because a large degree of bone loss is required – typically between 30% and 40% – before osteopenia can be identified radiologically. Although X-rays will detect moderate or severe fractures, subtle deformities may be difficult to identify and diagnose: in any event, in about 25% of fracture cases the BMD is not low and there is no particular risk of secondary fractures. This is why other radiological techniques have been developed for the investigation of osteoporosis (see Diagnostic Focus, above).

The pattern of trabecular bone and the thickness of cortical bone can be assessed using serial measurements from a number of identical dated planar X-rays. Quantitative methods of distinguishing between the various stages of bone loss have been proposed, but there is no available means of defining the degree of porosity of the cortical bone. Using X-ray, it is possible to highlight the opacity of the calcium phosphate of bone, but these X-rays do not identify the cause of the osteopenia.

The use of planar X-rays in making comparisons and taking accurate measurements is complicated by the variability in the process of producing X-ray films. These variations include the reduction with time in X-ray power from the source, the uneven emission of X-rays from the source, causing variable exposure of the film, and loss of strength over time of the developing chemical agents that are used to process the film. In order to combat these inconsistencies, standard reference objects can be used, such as the cadaveric metacarpal bone or an aluminium step wedge.

Radiological techniques for specific skeletal areas

Back bone

The gradual change in the shape of the individual vertebrae of the spine, which progresses from end plate collapse to wedge formation and eventually crush fracture, is brought about by the loss of bone mass. As bone density is reduced, the vertebrae gradually lose their opacity when viewed under X-rays. Osteoporosis of the spine is caused by the loss of bone mass from the centre of the vertebrae, whilst the outer cortical bone layer remains intact. This is brought about initially by the loss of horizontal trabeculae, causing the vertical trabeculae to become more distinct; with further loss, the vertebrae become increasingly hollow. In order to classify the amount of bone loss with the progression of the disease, a number of scales have been drawn up. These scales are used to identify the severity of osteoporosis by examining the X-ray appearance of the spine (see Diagnostic Focus, below).

The effect of osteoporosis on the spine tends to lead to a gradual curvature, which can be seen as a loss of height; this evidence can be used as an index of bone loss. Further detailed measurements of vertebrae, including the ratio of the central disc height to central vertebral body height, from sections of the lumbar and lower thoracic spine, may be made to produce a more accurate comparison over time. This measurement is dependent upon the relative change in the shape of the discs and the vertebral plates; the discs expand and are heightened, while the vertebrae are reduced as they are softened by the lack of trabeculae and reshaped by the expanding discs to a biconcave shape. If a vertebra is excessively distorted into a wedge shape, then that vertebra has to be discounted; similarly, if a vertebra should form an asymmetrical wedge shape, measurement will prove difficult and unreliable.

A change in vertebral outline is not exclusive to osteoporosis, in fact it is more common following trauma, particularly in young healthy

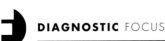

Classification of vertebral deformity (T4–L5) using a spine index	
Index	Description of vertebrae T4–L5
0	No signs of osteoporosis
1	Increased radiolucency
2	Infraction of one end plate
3	Infraction of both end plates Severe biconcavity Wedged vertebra
4	Compression fracture
Spine index	Sum of the indices of the vertebrae T4–L5

adults, where it is not related to loss of bone mass. This is certainly the case in the discovery of a single wedge-shaped vertebra; but should there be two or more compressed vertebrae, then this is more than likely to be related to a low bone mass.[3]

Hip bone

Another crucial part of the skeleton that has been identified as being important as a predictor of bone mass is the head of the femoral bone. An index has been developed based on the density of trabecular bundles within the head of the femoral bone measured with planar X-ray and using reference standards to maintain a set calibration of all the grades. In the application of this index it has been observed that patients presenting with a fracture are often classified as having an expected normal bone density value. Therefore, this index, although helpful in epidemiological studies, is not as useful when applied to the individual patient. Similarly, the measurement of the thickness of the calcar femorale, which was thought to be a reliable predictor of the risk of a fractured neck of femur has been found in clinical use to be inadequate when applied to the individual.[3]

Peripheral bone

The thickness of cortical bone in the hand can be measured easily and accurately by using planar X-rays, since the metacarpal bone consists of cortical bone only. Fine-grain non-screen postero-anterior X-ray films of the hands are taken, using a standard distance between the hand and X-ray tube-film to eliminate errors in repeated assessments. A calculation is then made to assess the total volume of cortical bone, which gives a precise picture of the volume of bone present. This method of measurement is limited in its clinical application, because it is only applicable to peripheral sites and cannot be transposed onto more critical areas, such as the spine or hip where there is a greater content of trabecular bone.

The method employed to ascertain the thickness of the cortical bone is to measure the total width of the metacarpal bone, usually using the second metacarpal bone, although accuracy can be improved by using the third and fourth metacarpal bones of both hands. Measurements are made using fine needlepoint vernier callipers on X-ray films of each hand at different points in time. In order to limit inter-observer errors, it is important to employ the same observer throughout the process.

Having carried out the necessary measurements from the X-rays, the observer must convert these measurements into an estimation of total bone density. At present, the conversion of the width of the metacarpal bone to a volume of bone relies on a number of assumptions; namely, that the metacarpal bone is like a perfect cylinder, the length of the metacarpal bone or surface area can be used to correct for body size and any variations in measurements are dependent on the skill of the observer. This makes the accuracy of these calculations of limited value as it is difficult to control for these variables. Cortical bone, when measured in this way, has been found to provide the most accurate estimate of bone mass, when compared with that derived from ash weight of cremated bodies.

The manner of bone growth and the changes that occur in development are easily monitored by metacarpal X-rays; but once bone has matured and is remodelling itself within the Haversian systems, becoming subject to age-related bone loss, the process cannot be monitored by the metacarpal measurement of cortical bone. This is because the cause of age-related fractures is the loss of strength from the bone due to depletion of trabecular bone, rather than loss of cortical bone, and the metacarpal bone cannot predict this.

The assessment of bone mass using X-rays of metacarpal bones is a simple, fast, cheap and safe method, but although there is some possible correlation between age-related loss of bone mass and metacarpal cortical bone size, the technique has many drawbacks, which have led to other methods of bone mass measurement being tried.

Conventional X-rays can only detect bone damage that has already taken place and are therefore poor predictors of future outcomes, unless the deterioration of the bone is significant. Clearly there is need for a more sensitive test that can be used as a diagnostic tool for osteoporosis.[3]

Photodensitometry

In photodensitometry an X-ray film, usually of the distal ulna, proximal radius and the metacarpal bones, is taken and placed between a light source and a photoelectrical cell, which has been calibrated. Readings are then taken, giving a value to the density of the measured bone. This technique is limited to these particular bones, since they are not affected by soft tissue shadowing, which excludes the use of other more deep-seated bones. Because of the lack of reproducibility of planar X-rays, together with other variations and inaccuracies, this method has limited scope and has become obsolete following the development of more sophisticated instruments.[3]

Photon absorptiometry

Photon absorptiometry involves the use of a radioactive isotope that emits a pure source of monochromatic radiation at a defined strength. This is attenuated by objects in its path, such as bone or soft tissue, and the resulting amount of attenuation is then measured by a detector. Photon absorptiometry is available as a single or dual beam of radiation.

The photon beam will measure the total bone mineral content of all the bone in its path; it does not differentiate between cortical and trabecular bone. Although photon absorptiometry cannot supply information regarding the growing bone, its unique advantage over planar X-rays is that it can detect changes in bone mineral density in cortical bone. The advantages of photon absorptiometry are listed in the Diagnostic Focus below.

DIAGNOSTIC FOCUS

Advantages of photon absorptiometry
Uniform intensity of the beam
Little scattering of radiation because of the narrowness of the beam
Monoenergetic radiation which reduces the selective filtration of the beam by the tissue

Single-beam photon absorptiometry

The single-beam photon absorptiometry (SPA), which has been available for over 30 years, uses a highly collimated beam of radiation, normally from iodine-125. This beam is allowed to pass through a limb and the resultant radiation intensity is measured by a collimated scintillation counter.

This method of measuring bone mineral density relies on scanning a unit length of a limb. This is then compared with a predetermined standard and a calculation is made based on skeletal size. The result is quoted as a density per unit area. The normal site used is the distal radius, and in order to render the scanning reproducible, a sequence of parallel scans are carried out along the arm. The distal radius provides the best site, being 70% trabecular bone, and would establish a sound correlation for the whole body, whereas the midpoint of the radius is cortical bone and the os calcis is mainly trabecular bone.

These measurements of isolated bones do not predict the risk of fracture at the femoral neck or foresee the possibility of vertebral fractures within the spine. However, the technique of single photon absorptiometry is relatively simple and cheap so it is ideal for identifying people with a low level of cortical bone or inadequate bone mass and for monitoring those found to be at risk, since it is possible to repeat this process. Further work on this technique in order to improve results led to the development of dual photon absorptiometry, which has largely surpassed single photon absorptiometry and become the gold standard method of choice.[4]

Dual photon absorptiometry

Dual photon absorptiometry requires two different sources of radiation, emitted at different energy levels. In the past, this has meant using two isotopes of different elements, the usual choices being from iodine-125, americium-241 and caesium-137. More recently, however, gadolinium-153 has become the isotope of choice, because it emits radiation at two energy levels, namely 42 and 100 keV. This is perfect for measuring bone density at deep-seated sites, which are surrounded by soft tissue, such as the femoral neck and the spine. The gadolinium-153 isotope has a half-life of 242 days with a useful active life of 12–18 months, when the source can be said to be uniform. The disadvantage of using gadolinium-153 is that it is difficult to source and hence expensive.

The dual-energy X-ray absorptiometry (DEXA) scanner has become the best instrument currently available for the measurement of bone mineral density, but it must be precisely located over the site of investigation in order to ensure reproducibility. The scanner converts the measurement of the bone mineral density into an equivalent mass of the hydroxyapatite that is present. The accuracy of this method is extremely high, the resulting error rate being between 1 and 4%, but if the radioactive source is altered during an observation period, it is then necessary to recalibrate the scanner in order to maintain the uniformity of the results.[5]

The DEXA scanner works by emitting two different photon energy X-rays and then measuring the received transmission; the difference between the two can be defined as the density of the object. It is capable of measuring accurately, precisely and at a much-reduced X-ray dose, the density of the bone mass at various sites in the body, including the lumbar vertebrae, hip and wrist areas.

Although the DEXA scanner is now looked upon as the main diagnostic tool in detecting any underlying osteoporosis, it does have limitations:

- It measures only the mineral content of the bone, which is then converted into a BMD, this may give a higher bone mass in the presence of osteomalacia.
- It will give false readings when certain conditions already exist: for instance, in the presence of vascular calcification, degenerative discogenic and paravertebral disease. The use of contrast media may also alter measurements of spinal scans, particularly in the elderly.
- It may not provide a detailed enough interpretation where variables in body/skeletal size or previous fractures or deformities exist.
- It will not detect variations in the amount of soft tissue surrounding the skeleton, especially when there is an uneven distribution of fat; this could give a false reading of the BMD.
- Its successful use is dependent on minimising or the elimination of human error.
- There is a need to calibrate the scanner according to the cohort of the population being tested, rather than on data based on different people from other racial mixes.
- The scanner has a high initial cost and a high maintenance cost, because the radioactive source is expensive and difficult to obtain.
- A single scan can last up to 30 minutes, rendering it impracticable as a screening tool to be used in studies involving large numbers of the population.

These limitations have prompted researchers to look for the most suitable method of determining the optimum site at which to measure the BMD; this has now been focused upon the hip, and the most pertinent reading is of the BMD of the total hip bone.[6]

Quantitative computer tomography

Quantitative computer tomography (QCT) is a means of measuring a true volumetric density following modification. QCT can enable the investigator to differentiate between trabecular bone and cortical bone of the spine, making it a more specific technique in identifying early bone loss.

QCT produces a three-dimensional picture of the bone being measured and is easily replicated, yielding a low error rate of between 1 and 3%, but it requires a great deal of skill on the part of the operator to master the technique. The use of this system has been tested on tibia and femoral shaft; use at other sites poses a problem because of the difficulty of overcoming the effect of attenuation of surrounding soft tissue, in comparison with the attenuation of the bones. This method is of limited use in the measurement of limb and peripheral bones and even spinal measurements are problematical because of the increase in bone marrow fat that occurs with age, which affects the resolution of the instrumentation. Presently QCT cannot be used to measure BMD of the hip. Moreover, it employs a greater dose of radiation than the DEXA scanner, making it unsuitable for repeated use in further monitoring.[7]

Radioisotopes

By measuring the uptake of radiolabelled isotopes of bisphosphonates into the bone, it is possible to measure, via the hydroxyapatite crystals, the level of activity in the bone, particularly bone turnover. This technique is useful where there is a need to identify abnormal metabolic activity within the bone, as in Paget's disease, and where multiple lesions exist as a result of invasive metastatic bone cancer. Although the use of radioactive isotopes will show the effects of osteoporosis over a reasonable time scale, normally extending over a year, the technique is more important in determining the root cause of a condition; that is, whether it is osteoporosis or an alternative diagnosis.[8]

Portable devices

The BMD of the peripheral skeleton can be read accurately with the use of either single photon absorptiometry or single-energy X-ray absorptiometry (SXA), normally of the forearm. Portable devices using these techniques are widely available and relatively easy to use, but quality control must be stringently monitored in order to obtain precise measurements. However, the use of SPA or SXA may not yield an accurate prediction of hip or spinal BMD. Recently, the development of peripheral DEXA and QCT in a portable scanner has led to their increased use in similar situations.

Ultrasound measurements

Ultrasound is used in a variety of ways to investigate and predict fracture risk, either as a single technique or in combination with others. Ultrasound has the advantage over densitometry in that the structure of the bone can be examined and the differences between fragility factors and degenerative damage distinguished. Ultrasound can be of benefit in the diagnosis of the elderly who have some bone loss by defining their risk of fracture. In this way ultrasound can be used at various peripheral sites of the body in helping both to confirm diagnosis and to predict the likelihood of impending fractures.

Conclusion

Currently, there is some debate regarding the diagnostic technique that is best suited to the diagnosis of osteoporosis. Certainly the DEXA scanner provides the most appropriate measurements at the critical sites of the body, but it does have its disadvantages, as explained earlier. There is clearly a need for standardisation of the various techniques and an algorithmic approach to the process of diagnosis. Ultimately, the choice of the test used depends on the availability of the equipment. The development of more practical and portable devices will lead to the wider availability of a range of techniques that can then be used in combination to further define the risk of bone loss.[9]

Biochemical markers

Biochemical tests are used in a number of ways to confirm the underlying cause of osteoporosis and to determine useful interventions in both prevention and treatment. These tests involve the assessment of calcium levels and the identification of the rate of bone turnover.

First, calcium and phosphate serum levels should be measured to discover if the cause of the osteoporosis is the natural ageing process or if the disease is complicated by either deficiencies of calcium, vitamin D, parathyroid hormone or malabsorption and poor metabolism of essential nutrients. Tests should be undertaken to isolate the particular deficiency, which must then be remedied, in order to discover if this reverses the changes associated with osteoporosis.

Calcium

Calcium exists in the body both in a free form and bound to the plasma protein albumin. Therefore, the serum albumin level must be known. When the total calcium level can be calculated, this is termed the corrected calcium level.

Further examination of calcium can be carried out using the level obtained from a 24-hour urine collection. This is usually normal in osteoporotic patients, but a low level would indicate either poor calcium absorption from the intestine or a low dietary intake of calcium. A high level of calcium in the urine, hypercalciuria, would be indicative of high rate of absorption of calcium from the intestine, a lack of conservation of calcium by the kidney or an increased rate of bone resorption. Hypercalciuria frequently occurs as result of immobilisation, in conjunction with an increase in bone turnover. This could follow a fracture sustained during the early part of the menopause or in the young. The level of bone resorption is normally predicted by the level of calcium in the urine in the fasting state. This can be used to monitor the effectiveness of inhibitors of bone resorption when compared with the creatinine level. This test has now been superseded by the use of more specific biochemical markers of bone turnover, which provide a higher degree of accuracy.

Vitamin D

Now that it is possible to carry out individual tests to ascertain both deficiencies of vitamin D and the parathyroid hormone, both tests should be undertaken as a priority in order to establish a normal level. These deficiencies generally appear simultaneously. In vitamin D deficiency, not only is the serum level low, but the parathyroid hormone is high. This would suggest a vitamin D deficiency-induced secondary hyperparathyroidism.

Bone turnover

Biochemical markers of bone turnover can be divided into two different types: those that relate to bone formation and those that relate to bone resorption (see Diagnostic Focus, below).

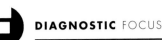

Biochemical markers of bone turnover

Bone formation	*Bone resorption*
Serum	**Serum**

Alkaline phosphatase (ALP)
    Total ALP
    Bone-specific ALP
	Tartrate-resistant acid phosphatase (TRAP)

	Pyridinoline/deoxypyridinoline C-telopeptide (ICPT)

Osteocalcin (OC)/bone gla
protein (BGP)
    Intact molecule
    Fragments	

Propeptides of type I collagen	
C-Terminal propeptide (NICP)	
N-Terminal propeptide (PINP)	
	Urine
	Pyridinoline/deoxypyridinoline
	Free (Pyrilink/Pyrilink-D)
	C-terminal telopeptides (CTX, Crosslaps)
	N-terminal telopeptides (NTX, Osteomark)
	Hydroxylysine glycosides
	Fasting urine calcium and hydroxyproline

Bone formation

The cells within the bone that form its structure are called osteoblasts; these cells arrange themselves in concentric circles and maintain the rigidity and strength of the bone. During bone formation the osteoblast must have a rich supply of minerals such as calcium and phosphorus. A number of proteins are also required to form the architecture of the bone, providing the bone strength. These proteins include bone-specific alkaline phosphatase, osteocalcin (OC) or bone Gla protein (BGP), as well as various derivatives of collagen. All of the aforementioned proteins have been used as biochemical markers of bone formation, particularly BGP, as it has a short half-life and undergoes a variation of between 15% and 20% throughout the day in a circadian rhythm. The measurement of BGP, either as the whole molecule or as the N-terminal–mid peptide, mimics other invasive indices of bone formation.

Bone resorption

The lack of a clear and accurate test to judge the amount of bone resorption occurring at any one time has inspired researchers to attempt a number of different assays of various proteins and peptides. For example, one test used fasting urine calcium and another test used hydroxyproline; neither proved accurate enough. Tests measuring hydroxylysine and tartrate-resistant acid phosphatase (TRAP) await further evaluation as to their specificity.

Meanwhile, the collagen derivatives and the telopeptides have been found to be the most appropriate biochemical markers for bone resorption, the results closely reflecting those of bone histology and calcium kinetic studies. In particular, pyridinoline (Pyr), deoxypyridinoline (D-Pyr) have been investigated to assess their ability to be released only during bone resorption; hence the production of immunoassays to detect free Pyr (Pyrilink) and free D-Pyr (Pyrilink D) in urine. The development of tests based on derivatives of these compounds, namely the C-terminal (CTX) and N-terminal (NTX) derivatives, are also available. These biochemical markers undergo dramatic variations throughout the day, which has led to a debate as to the optimum time and over how long a period urine should be collected for sampling.

Clinical uses

Although biochemical bone markers are primarily used to define the degree of bone formation and bone resorption, they can also be used to identify those patients who are at risk of rapid bone loss and fracture. Biochemical bone markers may be employed both as an aid to the choice of therapy and in its subsequent monitoring.[6]

Rapid bone loss

In general, bone loss during adult life is between 1% and 5% per year, as monitored using a DEXA scanner (which has a relative error rate of between 1% and 3%). This may not be significant enough to distinguish differences in an individual and between individuals. In women who are going through the menopause, the rate of bone loss suddenly increases by a factor of between two- and fourfold. Using a combination of DEXA scanner and simple markers – serum alkaline phosphatase, urinary calcium and hydroxyproline – a 50% reduction in BMD has been reported in menopausal women after a 12-year period. This would suggest that there are two different types of women, namely those who lose bone slowly and those who lose bone at a much faster rate. With improved bone markers, these differences could be detected earlier.

In elderly women, who may be at least 20 years postmenopausal, the rate of bone loss has been shown to decrease to the level prior to the menopause. This information was based on the evidence of clinical studies that looked at bone turnover at the cellular level, not at the skeletal level. In more recent studies, in which highly sensitive biochemical bone markers were employed, it was shown that the bone turnover throughout the skeleton varies considerably from individual to individual.[6]

Fracture risk

The probability of a fracture is dependent primarily on two factors: the BMD and the rate of bone loss. If a woman approaching the menopause does so with an established low BMD and this is coupled with a high rate of bone loss, then she will be at a much greater risk of suffering a spinal or hip fracture. As stated previously, the population can be divided into two main groups, one that loses bone mass quickly and the other that loses bone mass slowly. People who fall within the 'fast group' will develop the signs and symptoms of osteoporosis a great deal earlier in life than the 'slow losers'.

Because a one-off BMD measurement with a DEXA scanner will not distinguish between these two groups, BMD measurement should be combined with measurement of bone resorption using biochemical bone markers. When a high rate of bone resorption occurs this will lead to a reduction in strength, showing itself in two distinct ways. First, changes in the architecture of the bone will occur, with a reduction in the main structural trabecular bone. Secondly, bone resorption will take place faster than bone formation, causing a reduction in the total amount of bone. These changes, coupled with an overall reduction in BMD, could lead to a greater risk of hip fracture in the fast bone mass losers.

Monitoring therapy

Once treatment for osteoporosis has been commenced, it will normally take at least two years before changes in BMD will be observed on DEXA scanners. However, if biochemical bone markers are employed, any change in bone formation and resorption will be seen after a period of between three and six months. This demonstrates the importance of the role that these bone markers play in demonstrating a response to therapy at a much earlier stage.

Choice of therapy

In some clinical studies it has been shown that the aim and choice of therapy will be dictated by the category of bone mass loser (fast or slow) into which the patient falls. For instance, in a patient who is a fast bone loser, anti-resorption therapy would be best, whereas in a slow bone loser, the bone formation therapy would be more appropriate. Bone markers may be used to judge the optimum time period for each therapy.

Limitations

The main limitation of biochemical bone markers is that they can only give information on the whole skeleton; unlike the DEXA scanner, they cannot identify any particular areas of weakness. Also, there are neither national nor international agreed standards for these markers because of the difficulty in reproducing results. There can be as much as between 5% and 10% variation in serum markers, and the urine-derived bone markers can differ by up to 35%. These variations in assays make any useful assessment of individuals very difficult. Clearly, work must continue to discover the most viable method of assay, or a means by which the variations can be minimised with correlation to other tests, such as creatinine excretion with urinary telopeptides.

A number of the biochemical markers follow a circadian rhythm, which creates a problem regarding the best time to collect the sample. Differences in liver and kidney function will lead to differences in the speed of metabolism and excretion, which is why attempts have been made to correct for creatinine clearance (a measure of kidney function).

In conclusion, the use of the biochemical markers must be placed in context and care used in the choice of the most appropriate time to apply them. Clearly, their primary use is in assisting with the choice of therapy and its monitoring, rather than as a screening test. The particular bone marker chosen will depend on the local resources and the available expertise required to measure the results with a reasonable degree of accuracy and reproducibility.[6]

Bone biopsy

This is a simple orthopaedic operation in which a section of bone is removed using a bone chisel for microscopic examination. In order to obtain productive results for the investigation of osteoporosis, specific specimens are taken from a definitive bone site. Initially, the preferred site was the iliac crest, using an 8-mm core specimen of the whole bone, but there were often problems in obtaining a complete intact sample. This limited the value of the biopsy, as on some occasions only the cortical bone was obtained and the medulla and trabecular bone were absent because the sample broke off during the procedure. Also, the result from the iliac crest was not representative of a normal mature bone as it had been formed by ossification of the ligaments and cartilaginous metaplasia, rather than mineralisation of growing bone. In order to improve the technique and to procure a more representative assessment of mature bone, full-thickness transiliac biopsy is usually used today. This is taken through the wing of the ilium, into the space under the iliacus muscle, giving a sample of bone that is a cylinder of uniform size containing cortex–medulla–cortex.

Bone biopsy is used to identify the source of a metabolic bone disease, in order that an effective treatment plan may be started after a diagnosis has been ascertained. Possible diagnoses are osteomalacia, osteoporosis, hyperparathyroidism, Paget's disease and invasive metastatic bone disease. If bony metastatic disease is suspected, then X-rays should be carried out beforehand, in order to determine the most suitable site for the biopsy and to obtain the optimum result. A bone biopsy can be used to discover the histological structure of the bone and provides a means of identifying and quantifying the cellular components of mineralised and non-mineralised bone. The primary function of this procedure is to distinguish between osteoporosis and osteomalacia; other uses include the investigation of unexplained osteopenia that has not responded to therapy. Bone biopsies can also be used as a research tool to investigate the effect of experimental treatments carried out to improve bone structure, since up to four biopsies are possible.

The bone biopsy may be performed under local anaesthetic as an outpatient procedure or, in the case of an elderly patient at risk, an overnight stay may be recommended. A local anaesthetic, usually lidocaine (lignocaine) is given, often with a benzodiazepine sedative to act as an amnesiac, so that the patient has no recall of the procedure. Once the patient is anaesthetised, then the initial incision may begin, a passage is cleared to the bone and a bone biopsy instrument is introduced through the incision. The instrument is then inserted into the bone and note is taken, by the operator, of the resistance felt, as this will give a clue as to the nature of the bone: either resistant and healthy or soft because of osteoporosis or osteomalacia.[3]

References

1.   Royal College of Physicians. *Osteoporosis. Clinical Guidelines for Prevention and Treatment.* London: Royal College of Physicians, 1999.
2.   Dixon A S, Hawkins S, Williams C. Circadian variation in segmental vertebral height in spinal osteoporosis. *Osteoporosis* I.
3.   Woolf A D, Dixon A S. *Osteoporosis: a Clinical Guide.* London: Martin Dunitz, 1988.
4.   Mazess R B. Estimation of bone and skeletal weight by direct photon absorptiometry. *Invest Radiol* 1971; **6**: 52–60.
5.   Dunn W L, Heinz M S, Wahner H W, *et al.* Measurement of bone mineral content in human vertebrae and hip by dual photon absorptiometry. *Radiology* 1980; **136**: 485–487.
6.   South African Medical Association – Osteoporosis Working Group. Osteoporosis clinical guideline. *S Afr Med J* 2000; **90**: 907–944.
7.   Mazess R B. Errors in measuring trabecular bone by computed tomography due to marrow and bone composition. *Calcif Tissue Int* 1983; **35**: 148.
8.   Fogelman I, Bessent R G, Cohen H N, *et al.* Skeletal uptake of diphosphonate-method of prediction of postmenopausal osteoporosis. *Lancet* 1980; **2**: 667–670.
9.   Langton C, Palmer S B, Porter R W. The measurement of broadband ultrasonic attenuation in cancellous bone. *Eng Med* 1984; **13**: 89.

6

Clinical interventions

In an ideal world, all people in the relevant categories would be screened for osteoporosis, the decision to screen someone being based on certain risk factors or the outcome of a specific diagnostic test. The result of these techniques would decide whether or not treatment would be offered or provided. As this is not realistically possible, the decision to treat will be based on the ability to determine a definitive diagnosis triggered by the following considerations:

- the nature of the disease
- the patient profile
- the efficacy and cost of available treatment.

The decision whether or not to make a clinical intervention in osteoporosis will be influenced by the probability of a fracture occurring. The fracture is then the reason for the diagnosis. Otherwise, as with any other condition, clinical risk factors would be established in order to define the possibility of a person's developing the disease and/or its consequences; this prognosis would be based either on a specific diagnostic test, or by establishing which clinical presentations would predict the likelihood of the disease.[1]

In earlier chapters we have seen that the present condition of the bones can be defined by measurement of bone mass density (BMD) and calculating by how many standard deviations the BMD differs from the normal. This does not, however, present the complete picture, as there are other predisposing factors to be taken into account, such as the patient's lifestyle and level of physical activity. Two individuals with identical BMD measurements will have the same underlying bone strength but, depending on clinical risk factors, their risks of developing established osteoporosis may be completely different.

In practice, the presence and the severity of clinical risk factors will often lead to clinical interventions that take the role of prophylaxis of either a primary or a secondary fracture. These clinical interventions may well be instituted prior to a bone mass measurement being carried out; this may be due to the lack of availability of facilities and the cost of performing the diagnostic test. Restrictions on the access to these bone mass measurements limit both the number of follow-up tests and the monitoring of any current treatment.

Clinical risk factors can be classified into two separate categories: those that are patient-based, such as lifestyle factors, and those that are disease-based, for instance the severity or incidence of symptoms. Opinions differ regarding the relative importance and weighting that should be placed on each clinical risk factor, particularly where patient-based factors are concerned. The presence of a fragility fracture is the most significant indication that would lead to automatic consideration of therapeutic intervention. Other factors deal with the potential to prevent fractures; the consequential loss of mobility, impoverished quality of life and morbidity that may follow.

Further discussion of the clinical risk factors with regard to the specific type and significance of each will be dealt with in more detail when looking at the possible development of a screening programme (Chapter 12). In considering the nature of the clinical intervention, a major controlling factor will be the degree to which the disease has become established on presentation. This will, in turn, have a bearing on the type and level of intervention required to restore the patient to as near as possible a normal state of health. The achievement of the desired outcome will depend on the potential for improving the overall quality of life.

In order to describe the various clinical interventions these have been divided into the two separate categories in which the treatment is usually provided, by different clinical specialities, namely the medical and the surgical.

Medical interventions for osteoporosis

Medical treatments for osteoporosis consist of the various drug treatments used to prevent further damage to the bone structure by maintaining the integral bone strength. The choice of agent depends on the condition of the bone and the degree of bone loss that has occurred in comparison with the predicted peak bone mass. Any underlying processes must be identified at the same time as the diagnosis is made, otherwise the chosen treatment will not have the expected effect, the patient will not improve and in certain circumstances, bone loss may be accelerated.

Sources of bone loss

The most common cause of bone loss in women is a reduction in sex hormone secretion brought about by the menopause. This can be either natural as part of the ageing process or induced as a result of surgical removal of the uterus (hysterectomy) with or without removal of the ovaries (oophorectomy). The surgical menopause can produce a marked reduction in bone loss, greater than that sustained from a natural menopause. A hysterectomy on its own will have some effect on bone loss, even if the ovaries are left in place, as there is an inevitable reduction in ovarian function, which may be related to surgical effects on the blood supply of the ovaries. Even the manipulation of the fallopian tubules, such as ligation or application of clips for sterilisation, can affect the release of oestrogen from the ovaries. All women who have had these procedures should be assessed as to the likelihood of their developing osteoporosis and being at risk of fracture.

Although men do not undergo a similar loss of androgens from a process such as the menopause, there is a gradual decline in the release of androgens with age. This is not seen as a risk factor for either osteoporosis or related fractures. However, men who have experienced a dramatic loss of androgens, such as following a surgical or a medical castration for prostate or testicular cancer, do undergo an alteration in their skeletal architecture due to a loss of bone mass. The changes in the male skeleton from the loss of androgens mimic the effects seen in women after the menopause.

In both sexes there is a gradual loss of bone mass with age once peak bone mass has been achieved. Although on average men have a higher bone mass than women, the rate of bone loss with age is the same in the sexes, except in perimenopausal women, when bone loss is rapid. In general, the risk of osteoporosis and subsequent fractures is greater with age and it is known that the incidence of fractures, particularly the neck of the femur, is greatest in people over the age of 80.

Deficiency diseases

The development of a deficiency disease is normally due to the absence of essential nutrients from the diet; this is especially seen during the growing period when there is an increased demand for all of these essential nutrients. Historically, it was in childhood that bone deficiency diseases became apparent. Children growing up with inadequate diets and poor housing developed with malformed limbs, unable to provide the structural support required to perform the normal movements of an active life.

The major deficiency disease of past generations was caused by lack of vitamin D. This led to osteomalacia, a softening of bones, commonly known as rickets, which was prevalent in many northern European cities in the nineteenth century. Rickets was widespread in such communities because possible exposure to sunlight was limited due to the sparse number of days of sunshine and the inability of sunlight to penetrate into streets with tall buildings either side. This became an increasing problem in the early part of the twentieth century, when more and more people were living in cities, within dwellings that were built very close together, providing cheap housing for the workforce of the industrial nations. The consequence of this environment was that children were growing up unable to join the industrial workforce as they were incapable of doing the physical work demanded because of the strictures of their bone deformities. Therefore, in the light of the problem, the government of the day decided to step in and ensure that everyone obtained sufficient vitamin D by passing a law that certain essential foods should be fortified with this vitamin. Thus, bakers were instructed to fortify white bread with vitamin D and manufacturers of margarine were obliged to add vitamin D to their products.

These measures have largely eliminated rickets as a childhood illness in the UK, and it is now seen only occasionally in the older immigrant population. The reason that the immigrant population is more susceptible to vitamin D deficiency is that they are accustomed to dressing in a fashion to ward off the effects of strong sunlight and to remaining indoors while the sun is at its height. In temperate countries, the sun is neither so strong nor the hours of sunlight so long as to warrant such restrictions on either dress or behaviour.

Another cause of vitamin D deficiency in immigrant populations is the tendency to follow a diet that lacks foods containing vitamin D. This deficiency can lead to osteomalacia and bone deformities. If such conditions are discovered early enough, then a course of ultraviolet therapy will help to boost stores of vitamin D, and to some degree correct, the initial stages of bone abnormalities. This problem has increased to such an extent within the Asian immigrant population, that health promotion programmes specifically targeting Asian communities have been developed in many areas.

Problems created by a lack of vitamin D are compounded when calcium, another essential nutrient, fails to be consumed in adequate quantities. Calcium is essential during the early years to ensure the development of healthy teeth and good strong bones. It was deemed important enough in the diet of children to warrant the provision of free school milk to all school-age children – up to the age of 12 years – in Britain. As this practice was stopped in the early 1970s, it is as yet too early to know whether this has had an adverse effect on public health, as it will be at least another 10 years before these children reach an age, at which the effects of osteoporosis are likely to become apparent.

These clinical interventions by government can be seen as public health initiatives to improve and to promote the enjoyment of good health by the whole of the population while reducing the incidence of preventable diseases. In the case of vitamin D, the fortification of general foodstuffs has almost eliminated rickets, with very little effect on people's daily lives or on the food they eat. The cost of this measure has been borne by the manufacturers, who have taken this into account in their pricing structure, since fortified bread is cheaper than its whole-meal equivalent, which contains sufficient vitamin D. This has meant that those patients who require information and treatment can be targeted, as statistics have shown that they are more likely to come from a certain proportion of the population. This is evidence of a government intervention designed to improve the health of the whole population and in this way to ensure that the developing workforce will be healthier and more able to fulfil manual work.[2]

Mineral supplementation

In comparing an expected peak bone mass with a reducing bone mass in the initial stages of osteoporosis, from whatever cause, the aim of therapy should be to increase bone formation. The first step in the role of assisting the improvement of bone formation is to ensure that there is sufficient substrate to enable this to take place. This will necessitate dietary assessment, particularly with regard to the content of the various minerals, including calcium, magnesium and phosphate, in the diet. Should there be any deficiencies then either the diet should be modified or supplements given (see Supplement Focus, below).[2]

Calcium

The element in the highest concentration within bone is known to be calcium. However, the main problem in the treatment of osteoporosis is how to improve the level of absorption; consequently, considerable thought has been expended on this subject. The achievement of a greater

Essential minerals required in the diet for bone formation (listed in the order of occurrence with the highest concentration first)
Calcium – the major element in bone
Phosphate – second most abundant element in bone
Sodium – high intake reduces bone growth
Boron – trace amount required
Silicon – trace amount required
Zinc – trace amount required

degree of calcium absorption invariably results in the recommended dose being far higher than that which would have been expected to be used in conditions relating to such a deficiency. Calcium absorption is influenced by the level of vitamin D, which is necessary not only for absorption itself but also for the uptake into bone. Thus, the use of calcium supplements is generally accompanied by vitamin D in order to enhance the effectiveness of the therapy in producing increasing bone formation.[2]

Phosphate

The second most abundant element in bone is phosphorus. Phosphorus is required in sufficient quantities to enable bone to form correctly, but if the diet is too high in phosphate then this can induce a secondary hyperparathyroidism and hypercalciuria. In the short term this may affect bone remodelling, but it is not thought to affect peak bone mass. The long-term consequences on the risk of osteoporosis are as yet unknown.[2]

Sodium

Although sodium does not have a direct effect on bone growth, a high sodium intake will cause an increase in calcium excretion. It is not known what effect this could have on bone metabolism. There is some evidence of an increase in bone turnover markers, namely hydroxyproline, but in population studies this has not been proved to affect bone mass. This could pose a problem for patients whose long-term diet includes a high sodium content but inadequate calcium.[2]

SUPPLEMENT FOCUS

Vitamins necessary for bone growth
Vitamin D – essential for calcium uptake and bone formation
Vitamin B_6 – cofactor for normal collagen metabolism
Vitamin B_{12}
Vitamin C – cofactor for normal collagen metabolism
Vitamin K

Vitamin D

It is known that a lack of vitamin D leads to the development of osteo-malacia, which, if allowed to continue, will cause deformity and fracture. It has also been observed that a low-grade deficiency of vitamin D produces a compensatory secondary hyperparathyroidism, which has the effect of increasing bone turnover, leading to osteoporosis. In order to increase bone formation supplementation with vitamin D in the presence of adequate calcium may be necessary (as detailed above).

Other essential nutrients

There are a number of other vitamins (see Supplement Focus, above) and minerals known to affect bone mass. These are: boron, silicon, zinc, vitamin B_6, vitamin B_{12}, vitamin C and vitamin K. Of these vitamin C and vitamin B_6 are required as cofactors for normal collagen metabolism and, if lacking, can precipitate osteoporosis.[2]

Hormone replacement therapy

The use of female sex hormones as a replacement therapy during the menopause has traditionally been employed to control the symptoms of the menopause. Initially, oestrogen only was prescribed, but now, more often than not, this is given in conjunction with progesterone. Oestrogen is an anti-resorptive agent that maintains bone resorption at a rate close to that in existence prior to the menopause. In some cases this can lead to an increase in bone mass. Hormone replacement therapy (HRT) thus helps to prevent rapid bone loss by reducing the increase in bone resorption that normally occurs during and after the menopause. The medications involved have evolved into a number of different pharmaceutical preparations and further developments have led to the inclusion of a more selective therapy, which has a reduced incidence of side effects.[3]

Other endocrine conditions

Although there is widespread awareness of the role of oestrogen deficiency as a cause of osteoporosis, there are other endocrine conditions which, if left untreated, can lead to osteoporosis. These are listed in the Risk Factor Focus below. There are specific treatments available for all these conditions that may prevent the progression to osteoporosis.

Primary hyperparathyroidism

This is a relatively common condition, affecting around one in a thousand people in the UK, in which too much parathyroid hormone is secreted by the parathyroid glands and the level of calcium in the blood rises (hypercalcaemia). In about 85% of cases it is caused by the presence of a single chief cell adenoma in one of the four parathyroid glands. This condition typically occurs in women who have just gone through the menopause, which suggests that a reduction in the level of oestrogen and/or progesterone could be responsible. By using oestrogen and progesterone it was hoped to discover whether women given HRT showed a reduction in calcium serum levels. This deficiency could be due to the direct effect of the HRT on the bone or on the secretion of the parathyroid hormone.

The result of primary hyperparathyroidism is that there is an increase in bone remodelling, which causes an increase in bone turnover with a resultant loss of bone mass. The bone mass is mainly lost from the limb bones and the spinal cord in a manner that seems to preserve

RISK FACTOR FOCUS

Endocrine conditions that can induce osteoporosis if uncontrolled
Primary hyperparathyroidism
Thyroid disease
Cushing's syndrome
Diabetes mellitus

bone strength, as has been identified from various studies, suggesting that trabecular bone remains intact with loss of the surrounding cortical bone. This indicates that if the bone mass can be restored through corrective surgery, by removing an overactive parathyroid gland, the bone will be able to return to the pre-diseased state. In practice it is found that the bone mass is gradually restored to former levels during the 12 months following surgery, and thereafter there is no further gain in bone mass. In a patient with a tendency to become osteoporotic, this results in the disease being particularly noticeable at the wrist bone.

Primary hyperparathyroidism is a mainly symptomless illness and is usually only picked up after a blood test identifies the hypercalcaemia. Further investigation using X-rays will show changes in some bones, especially in the fingers, arm and collarbones, with evidence of bone resorption in the skull. In severe cases of primary hyperparathyroidism, there is an increased risk of fractures, particularly of the vertebrae.

A definitive diagnosis of primary hyperparathyroidism comes from a high serum level of the parathyroid hormone, in conjunction with hypercalcaemia. The discovery of the hypercalcaemia, in most cases, would lead to further investigation in the form of a series of blood tests, one of which would be for parathyroid hormone.

As stated earlier, in the majority of cases, there is an adenoma of the parathyroid gland, which is usually removed surgically, along with a proportion of the parathyroid gland. The main contraindication occurs if the patient should prove unsuitable for a surgical procedure, because of adverse risks to health. In these patients, careful consideration should be given to balancing the benefits of surgery against the risks of the condition, if it is a mild form and the patient is asymptomatic. In such a case the necessity for continued monitoring will remain. In a patient with symptoms and severe hypercalcaemia who is not suitable for surgery, there may be some value in the use of a progestogen, for example norethisterone. Similarly, the bisphosphonates could be used to prevent further loss of bone mass, although they may not have a significant effect on the hypercalcaemia.[4]

Thyroid disease

In a patient with hyperthyroidism there is a raised rate of bone remodelling with further effects on bone turnover, as evidenced by increased levels of certain biochemical markers. Hyperthyroidism may cause an elevated level of calcium in the urine but only rarely has the same effect on calcium in the blood. If the level of thyroid hormone is raised over a period of years then osteoporosis will occur, probably caused by the direct action of the thyroid hormone on the bone.

If the hyperthyroidism occurs in later life then this will accelerate the gradual loss of bone mass that is part of the normal ageing process. The signs and symptoms of hyperthyroidism are few and non-specific; this is why the screening of thyroid function is common in the elderly.

Cushing's syndrome

This is a syndrome caused by an excessive release of glucocorticoids from the adrenal cortex, usually caused by an actively secreting tumour of the adrenals. It leads to the rapid development of osteoporosis and resultant fractures, usually of the spine rather than the limbs, such as the wrist or hip.

The usual treatment is to first find the source of the hypersecretion of the glucocorticoids. If it is a solid tumour of the adrenal gland, this can be removed surgically. If no single tumour can be isolated, then measures should be taken to reduce the function of the gland either by surgical excision of part of the tissue or by irradiation of the gland.[2]

Diabetes mellitus

There is some evidence that osteoporosis may be a problem in insulin-dependent diabetes mellitus, particularly in patients in whom the condition is poorly controlled. It is known that insulin-dependent diabetes is associated with low bone density but the changes that occur in the body composition of a diabetic make it difficult to obtain clear readings from a bone densitometry scanner. Therefore, possible changes in bone mineral density may be related to the influence of diabetes on the surrounding tissue rather than osteoporosis, although fractures have obviously taken place. The complications of diabetes can lead to poor eyesight and lack of balance, increasing the risk of a fall.[2]

Drug-induced osteoporosis

A number of drugs either affect bone metabolism or have an adverse effect on bone formation by reducing available nutrients. Often these drugs are given on a long-term basis and, if this is the case, consideration should be given to the possibility of osteoporosis. These effects should be counteracted by prescribing a modified dose or preventative

Drugs known to induce osteoporosis
Corticosteroids
Levothyroxine (thyroxine)
Anticonvulsants
Heparin
Lithium
Tamoxifen

therapy to reduce the side-effects.[2] Some of the drugs known to induce osteoporosis are listed in the Risk Factor Focus above.

Corticosteroids

Today, systemic corticosteroids are usually administered in a dose that is higher than physiological levels and sustained over a significantly long period – except when prescribed for certain common diseases. Corticosteroids are frequently administered in the form of repeated high-dose courses in order to reduce the symptoms of the underlying condition. Current knowledge would indicate that the adverse effect on the bone commences in the initial stages of the use of the corticosteroids; therefore, any preventative measures to be taken to reverse the damage should be initiated at the beginning of the therapy and not once the problem has arisen.

Corticosteroids directly affect the bone by suppressing the activity of osteoblasts, thus affecting bone remodelling and causing a reduction in the bone mineral content. The result is that the bone formed following remodelling is depleted in comparison with the original bone. Corticosteroids also create an indirect effect on bone by altering some of the endocrine functions; in particular, there is an increase in secretion of the parathyroid hormone. It is possible that this could be cause and effect as there is an increase in the serum calcium due to the losses from the bone.

The effect of corticosteroids on the other endocrine hormones may increase the risk of osteoporosis; for instance, corticosteroids influence sex hormone release, will induce Cushing's syndrome and may cause hypothyroidism and diabetes mellitus, all of which increase the risk of osteoporosis. Clearly, the use of corticosteroids needs to be monitored closely in order to detect any signs of adverse effects. If the length of the course is expected to be prolonged, then simultaneous prophylaxis with bisphosphonates would be advisable.[5]

Levothyroxine (thyroxine)

It is a well-established fact that one of the consequences of the ageing process is a decrease in the amount of thyroid hormone secreted. This leads to hypothyroidism. In order to treat this condition, supplements of levothyroxine (thyroxine) are often prescribed to compensate for the lack of the natural circulating hormone. If too much levothyroxine is given, then this will precipitate thyrotoxicosis, which is known to affect bone metabolism and increase the excretion of calcium. The effects on the skeleton are sufficient to encourage bone loss; this will be compounded by the existing bone loss due to the ageing process.

In the treatment of hypothyroidism, the effectiveness of the intervention is judged by the level of suppression of thyroid-stimulating hormone (TSH). If this is excessive, it will lead to a rapid loss of bone mass. Therefore, it is important when giving thyroid replacement therapy that the dose of levothyroxine is such that TSH levels remain within the normal range, as under- or over-dosing will create problems in the bone-metabolising process, leading to bone mass loss.

Anticonvulsants

A number of anticonvulsant drugs, such as phenytoin and carbamazepine, induce the activity of microsomal enzymes, promoting the metabolism of a number of nutrients, particularly vitamin D and its derivatives. The result of this is that normal dietary levels of vitamin D will be rendered ineffective, and the potential to absorb calcium from the gastrointestinal tract and uptake into the bone will be greatly reduced. In order to counteract this situation in the long-term, supplements of vitamin D to compensate for the increased metabolism are administered to patients taking these anticonvulsants.

Heparin

Administered over a prolonged period, heparin is known to induce osteoporosis, and in severe cases the use of this drug can lead to fractures. This observation is believed to be due to the direct effect of the heparin on the osteoclasts. Heparin is usually only prescribed either for prophylaxis or for treatment of a clotting disorder in pregnant women, when warfarin is contraindicated. It is thought that once the use of heparin is discontinued, the bone loss is restored, but this theory has yet to be tested over an extensive period. In recent years, the use of heparin has been superseded by the development of the low molecular weight heparins, although the effect of these on bone mass has still to be established.

Lithium

Continuous use of lithium over a number of years produces a rise in the secretion of the parathyroid hormone, with subsequent hypercalcaemia. This situation is compounded during the ageing process, resulting in an increased rate of bone mass loss, together with a reduced bone mineral content. This can be termed drug-induced hyperparathyroidism.

Tamoxifen

Tamoxifen is an oestrogen antagonist that is used in the secondary prevention and treatment of breast carcinoma, but it does have weak oestrogen agonist properties and is seen as a protective agent with respect to the skeleton in postmenopausal women. In premenopausal women it causes a reduction in bone mass, particularly at the spine and hip.

Drug treatments for osteoporosis

Apart from the drug treatment of any existing, underlying condition, there are just a few drugs that are indicated for the treatment of osteoporosis. The full description of these drugs and the manner in which they are used is given in the next chapter, but an introduction is included here to put the drugs within the context of an overall treatment plan in the fight against osteoporosis.

In the treatment of diagnosed osteoporosis, the first step is to ensure that the patient is following a diet that contains enough of the proper nutrients, in particular calcium and vitamin D. If these vitamins and minerals are not present in the daily meals in quantities large enough to compensate for the loss of bone, then either the diet should be altered to sustain these levels, or supplements must be given.

The next step depends on the sex of the individual; if female and postmenopausal, then HRT must be considered. This would be indicated for women who have a family history of osteoporosis, or who are subject to additional factors that increase the risk of osteoporosis. The duration of the treatment must be considered carefully, as in order to obtain maximum benefit, a five-year programme should be envisaged. This information ought to be explained in detail to the woman concerned as any adverse effects she is likely to suffer could limit or prohibit her use of the medication.

The only available active treatment for men is the bisphosphonates; these should be prescribed for men at risk of osteoporosis or who show early signs of the disease. In women, the bisphosphonates may be used either when HRT is not tolerated or when it is insufficient on its own to reverse the bone mass loss.[6]

Bisphosphonates

Initially used only in the treatment of hypercalcaemia, owing to their propensity to reduce the level of calcium in the blood, the first preparations of bisphosphonates were formulated as an injection, which needed to be given as a prolonged infusion because the active ingredients had poor solubility and required to be administered in a large volume infusion. Further developments ensued, following their use in some degenerative bone diseases, but it was not until an oral formulation was available, that their effectiveness against osteoporosis was discovered. The main problem arising from the oral preparations that are available is the lack of solubility, which limits the amount of the drug that can be absorbed. This is the source of a number of side effects.

Bisphosphonates have a direct effect on bone metabolism as they are taken up by bone and retained for a very long period in an inactive form. The reason for this is their strong affinity for the apatite crystals within the bone. Once bound to apaptite, the drugs become inactivated. The mechanism of action includes the reduction not only in number but also in activity of the osteoclasts. There is also an inhibitory effect on bone mineralisation. During the development of these drugs, it has become possible to heighten anti-resorptive effects, giving a subsequent reduction in bone mineralisation.

Surgical interventions for osteoporosis

The increase in fragility of bone in osteoporosis often first comes to light with the appearance of a fracture, either as a result of a low-impact

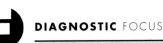

Main fractures associated with osteoporosis
Vertebral
Hip
Arm
Leg
Rib

injury or spontaneously, as in the case of a vertebral fracture (see Diagnostic Focus, above). At this stage, after a fracture has occurred, the bones are in a weakened state and the likelihood of a second fracture happening is much greater; therefore, any surgical intervention is limited because of the state of the damaged bones. The success of the surgical intervention will depend on the fracture sustained and any associated complications that could delay healing.

Common fractures sustained are of the wrist, hip and vertebrae. A wrist fracture sustained from a low-impact injury – usually occurring from an outstretched hand, trying to break a fall – may be the earliest indication of the condition. This type of fracture may not be the predicted displacement fracture, which is easily spotted on X-ray; but a more difficult to diagnose, hairline fracture. In both cases, the use of supportive care in the form of splints will allow the fracture to heal.[7]

Vertebral fracture

This is the most common fracture to occur in osteoporosis, often happening without any symptoms, causing the mildest of pain which may be thought to be from a previous injury. The absence of symptoms, with only transient changes, allows the problem to remain dormant and consequently unevaluated or noted on the patient's medical record. The incidence of vertebral fracture depends on the age and sex of the person. In a study, of patients between 70 and 75 years of age, 22% were found to have vertebral deformities, consistent with a previous fracture. Similarly, in a group of women aged from 54 to 73 years, 17% had evidence of vertebral fracture; over 50% of these, did not have a history of back pain.[8]

The majority of vertebral fractures happen as a result of everyday activities, rather than following any overexertion, and have even been known to occur whilst the person is lying down in bed. In other cases fractures follow falls from an upright position, road traffic accidents and bouts of strenuous activity. The initial fracture is frequently near the thoracolumbar junction, the mid-back. This manifests as a gradually increasing pain, felt either over a few days or – particularly after a fall – as a sharp pain. The pain radiates initially from the site of the fracture, but after a time may be spread over a greater area around the fracture.

If pain is present following a vertebral fracture then the patient will try to find the most comfortable position, which may be either lying down or sitting in a well-supported reclining chair. Muscle cramping or spasm often occurs as a complication of the fracture, and this can mask the source of the problem and may give rise to severe pain over a much larger area.

Following an acute vertebral fracture, particularly one originating from trauma, fragments of bone may become displaced. This is more common with compound fractures. In the worst scenario, most notably fractures of the thoracic spine, fragments can be posteriorly displaced into the spinal canal. This can lead to unilateral or bilateral signs of spinal compression, which must be fully investigated by magnetic resonance imaging (MRI). Spinal compression is a serious condition requiring surgical intervention, and will involve posterior stabilisation and anterior decompression of the fracture. In normal circumstances, a surgical operation will only be undertaken if the patient is fit enough to undergo a general anaesthetic, but in the case of a vertebral fracture where there is a high risk of neurological deficit, surgery will only be carried out in the presence of suspected cord compression.

In the absence of either nerve root or spinal cord compression healing of a spinal fracture will progress after the first few days. The symptoms of the fracture will diminish within the same timescale, usually resolving completely after about three months.

Treatment of the acute fracture will depend on where, in the spine, the fracture is located and this, in turn, will define the position in which the patient will feel most comfortable. Patients with lumbar spine fractures generally prefer to lie flat, with knees flexed, while patients with mid-thoracic fractures prefer to lie on one side, with a pillow to support the back. Bed rest is necessary for the first 2–7 days, after which mobilisation is considered as soon as possible, as prolonged bed rest will lead to muscular deconditioning and further bone loss.

Once the acute phase of treatment of the fracture has been completed, it is often found that rehabilitation can be hastened by the use of back supports. Initially this assistance might be in the form of lumbar support corsetry and extension braces. The use of such supports will depend on the patient's level of tolerance. If there is disease or any underlying back problem that affects the curvature of the spine, these supports, especially the wearing of extension braces, will be poorly tolerated. Lumbar support corsets and belts are more useful as aids to rehabilitation and will assist in increasing muscle strength. The belts are easy to use, comfortable and are helpful reminders to the patient to maintain good posture, since these appliances provide support without promoting disuse of the lower back musculature.[7]

Hip fracture

One of the most debilitating fractures caused by osteoporosis is that which occurs in the femoral neck of the hipbone. This can be either a transcervical or intertrochanteric fracture. Generally sustained in a fall, accompanied by an intense pain, these fractures have an immediate inhibiting effect on the patient's mobility and necessitate admission to hospital.

A dangerous situation arises when an elderly patient who is living alone has a fall and suffers such an injury. They may lie unattended and immobile for some hours before the alarm is raised and help summoned. This delay in the commencement of treatment can not only affect the fracture prognosis, but may also lead to the common complication of bronchopneumonia.

Treatment for hip fracture starts with the alleviation of the pain by the use of strong opioid analgesia, prior to emergency surgery. Diagnosis will be confirmed by a planar X-ray of the affected hip and pelvis to determine the site and extent of the fracture. Surgery consists of the repair of the fracture, either by pinning the bone or by total hip replacement. In the elderly, arthroplasty is the more successful treatment of choice and has been shown to speed recovery by shortening the period to mobilisation and to reduce mortality.[7]

Fractures of the arm

The elbow is frequently affected following a fall when the outstretched hand is used to reduce the impact; this action leads to an impacted subcapital fracture of the radius. In such cases, the elbow will show trauma, bruising and be painful but there will still be movement. Diagnosis can be confirmed by X-rays, then the fracture is allowed to heal by placing the affected limb in a sling to encourage the patient to rest it.

Fractures of the shoulder can be caused in a similar manner, producing a break of the proximal humerus. If the fracture is at the neck of the humerus, the results of surgical attempts at repair are often disappointing compared with those observed when the fragments are permitted to combine in the displaced position.[7]

Fractures of the leg

As well as fracture of the hip, there are a number of other fractures of the leg that can occur as a result of osteporosis. These include possible spontaneous metatarsal fracture, a stress fracture of the fibula and crush fractures of either tibial condyle. These fractures often occur because of the presence of rheumatoid arthritis, which produces a deformity of a joint, leading to a change in the weight distribution. Once the weight distribution has altered, the weight-bearing bones become stressed, causing the previously mentioned crush and stress fractures. In the case of the knee, a replacement arthroplasty will be necessary to realign the joint, prevent further damage and reduce the compression forces.[7]

Other fractures

Practically any bone within the skeleton may become fractured as a result of osteoporosis, but although fractures of the rib, tibia, arm and clavicle do occur and have been seen, these are rarely observed in osteoporotic patients.[7]

References

1. Royal College of Physicians. *Osteoporosis. Clinical Guidelines for Prevention and Treatment.* London: Royal College of Physicians, 1999.
2. Kanis J A. *Osteoporosis.* Oxford: Blackwell Science, 1996.
3. Prevention and treatment of osteoporosis. *MeReC Bull* 1994; **5**: 9–12.
4. Christiansen P, Steiniche T, Mosekilde L, *et al.* Primary hyperparathyroidism changes in trabecular bone remodelling. *Bone* 1990; **11**: 75–79.
5. Compston J E. Management of bone disease in patients on long term glucocorticoid. *Gut* 1999; **44**: 770–772.
6. Ferguson N. Osteoporosis prophylaxis and treatment. *Hospital Pharmacist* 2000; **7**: 69–71.
7. Woolf A D, Dixon A S. *Osteoporosis: a Clinical Guide.* London: Martin Dunitz, 1988.
8. Miller P D, McClung M. Prediction of fracture risk. *Am J Med Sci* 1996; **312**: 257–259.

7

Drug treatments

The underlying process in the development of osteoporosis is the gradual loss of bone mass, falling from the peak bone mass that is attained in early adult life between the ages of 25 and 30 years. The main factor that predicts the level of peak bone mass is genetic. This can be seen at all stages of development. As is the case for a number of diseases, a person's likelihood of developing osteoporosis has its origins in the genetic make-up of their parents. The first phase of development of bone mass is based on inherited factors, while the second phase, as the child grows up into late adolescence, requires the building blocks constructed from a good diet and plenty of exercise. The third phase is the maintenance of bone mass levels by taking a balanced diet of the correct vitamins and minerals, together with a reasonable level of exercise. The fourth and final phase is that of bone loss. It is only in this last phase that drug therapy will have an influence on bone development; this indicates that, important as drug therapy is, it plays only a minor role in comparison with the other major factors.[1]

Drug therapy for osteoporosis, whether for prophylaxis or treatment, is a relatively recent advance. The use and development of drugs has created a better understanding of how the condition arises and what is responsible for the underlying progress of the disease. Initial approaches to the use of medicines was from an elemental basis, either trying to replace what had been lost from the body or endeavouring to prevent that loss with dietary factors, such as increased calcium from dietary factors. It was not until the full extent and precise nature of the influence of the female sex hormones had been discovered that further exploration of the effect of supplementation was attempted. There was further research into other hormonal treatments before the specific drugs that have a direct effect on bone turnover were identified.

A number of drugs have been used in the prevention of osteoporosis. These fit into two broad categories: those that inhibit bone turnover and those that stimulate bone formation (see Management Focus, below). In normal bone, during the period of bone remodelling, there is a balance between bone formation and bone resorption, which

Drugs used in the treatment and prevention of osteoporosis

Inhibitors of bone turnover	Stimulators of bone formation
Oestrogens	Fluoride
Progestogens	Anabolic steroids
Calcitonin	Parathyroid hormone
Bisphosphonates	Intermittent calcitonin
Thiazide diuretics	
Calcium	
Vitamin D and its analogues	
Tibilone	
Raloxifene	

in adulthood maintains the bone mass at a reasonably constant level. In osteoporosis there is an imbalance whereby, at each remodelling site, the amount of bone that is formed does not keep pace with the quantity that is resorbed. Furthermore, in osteoporosis there is a reduction in bone turnover, decreasing the number of remodelling sites, although this does not compensate for the lack of bone formation.

The use of a drug to inhibit bone turnover will be seen at its most effective to increase bone mass, and at its least effective to maintain bone mass at a constant level, albeit of short duration. Any improvement in bone mass is slight and is not sustained for any length of time, as the results depend on the effect of the drug on the bone and the speed with which the bone can overcome the drug inhibition, to reach a new level of bone turnover. The reason for this is that inhibitors of bone turnover have the effect of reducing the amount of bone resorption by decreasing the number of new remodelling sites that are activated. However, at the existing remodelling sites, bone formation continues at the same pace although the level of bone resorption is diminished and, therefore, the overall bone mass will rise. The process of bone remodelling and, in particular, bone formation is a slow activity as tissue laid down in the bone becomes mineralised, to be incorporated as a fully functioning part of the bone. Therefore, the effectiveness of the drug will depend on its efficacy in inhibiting bone turnover and the level of bone mass loss

within the patient, prior to introduction of the drug. Under the influence of therapy, the skeleton will once more attempt to balance the two
functions of bone formation and bone resorption, but this time, in the
presence of an inhibitor, this process can extend over a period of two
years. Thus, any evaluation of the effectiveness of the drug should be
carried out at the end of this interval. Should any improvement be noted
at an earlier stage, for instance after one year, it should be realised that
these benefits may be only transient and may not be maintained over the
full two-year cycle.

If there are no changes in the balance of the dual processes of bone
formation and bone resorption throughout the cycle of bone turnover,
then this indicates that the bone is unaffected, except with regard to the
speed of each of these activities. The bone will then realign itself at the
lower rate of functioning, producing a reduced rate of bone mass loss.
In the longer term, the consequence of the use of these medications is a
slowing down of the rate of bone loss, rather than of the reversal of
skeletal bone losses, which is one reason why they are considered as preventative treatment rather than active treatment. In cases where patients
have a high bone turnover and yet a degree of bone mass increase is
experienced in the short term, this can be thought to be a reversing of
the existing bone mass loss; but as described previously, this result is not
continued in the longer term. Even though there may be only a slight
change in bone mass, the fact that the drug has reduced the rate of
decline of bone mass could prevent the patient's bone mineral density
reaching a level where an osteoporotic fracture is more or less inevitable.

It could be inferred that because of the effect the inhibitors have
on bone turnover, they provide an ideal solution to the problem of osteoporosis. As detailed above, inhibitors reduce bone loss and actually
increase bone mass; but the downside is that because of the reduction
in bone remodelling, fragility of the bone extends over a greater area.
Therefore, instead of a reduction in the number of fractures, an environment is created where fractures are more likely to occur because the
bone is failing to be renewed at the expected rate owing to the reduction of the remodelling sites. This is more liable to occur, when bone
remodelling has been eliminated entirely, whereas an incomplete inhibition of bone remodelling is deemed to be more advantageous. It is
important that the use of any drug treatment on the skeleton is monitored closely to investigate the direct effect on the bone in order to
ensure that the medication is having a beneficial effect.

The targeting of drug therapy to inhibit bone remodelling, which
takes place on the surface of the bone, could well succeed in increasing

bone mass, but may make no improvement in bone strength. The thickening of the bone surface increases cortical bone but does nothing to enhance the strength-providing trabecular bone, which may continue to lose mass at the same rate. Once trabecular bone is lost, it is not easily replaced because the osteoblasts are no longer attracted to the remnants of the bone; this makes the restoration of trabecular bone impossible.

An alternative method of reducing bone loss, in particular, loss of trabecular bone, would be the restriction of the resorption process, whereby cavities are created in the bone then repaired on a continuous basis. The normal depth of a cavity can extend across a third of the width of a trabecular bone; if the depth of these cavities were to be reduced, the likelihood of the complete erosion of the trabecular bone would be considerably diminished. Such an eventuality would promote the maintenance of both bone mass and bone strength, and thus reduce the risk of a fracture.[2–4]

Prevention

There are several different ways in which certain groups of drugs can be used in the prevention or treatment of osteoporosis; it is the distinction between these two aspects of the drugs that at times proves difficult. What may start as prevention of the condition will then alter with the passage of time to become treatment. As the disease progresses, the agent becomes active therapy. The dividing line between prevention and treatment is that normally prevention maintains the present state of health; but in osteoporosis the slow loss of bone mass is inevitable. Therefore, it is possible that a drug may fulfil either role, depending on the stage of the disease and the bone mass status of the patient.

In the initial stages of osteoporosis the aim is either to stop or to reduce the amount of bone loss from the skeleton. This can be achieved by improving the uptake of calcium into the bone or by trying to reverse the loss of calcium from the bone. Therapy can aim to intervene in the process of bone loss, altering the rate of bone metabolism to reduce bone turnover. The long-term purpose of all prevention is to reverse bone loss and increase bone mass; but most importantly to reduce the risk of a fracture by maintaining sufficient bone mass above the critical level, which, for each person, is different and has as yet to be defined. Therefore, once preventative drug treatments are introduced, close monitoring of the bone mass must be carried out, in order to detect any dramatic changes of bone mass.[3]

Calcium

The first attempts to mitigate bone loss involved the administration of calcium supplements to patients, the theory being that because these individuals were lacking in calcium they required extra dosage of this mineral. Initial studies showed that there appeared to be some merit in calcium supplementation, but further trials failed to emulate these first encouraging results. Besides, it was felt that as the subjects undergoing the tests were from a controlled environment they did not truly reflect the conditions that people experienced in everyday life.

Calcium is present to a greater or lesser extent in the diet and a number of other factors determine the amount of calcium that is eventually absorbed into the body's circulation and is available for uptake into the bone. It is well known that a diet high in calcium consumed during the developing years will help to ensure that peak bone mass is attained, and the possibility exists that it may even be exceeded. Continuing to follow a high calcium diet after peak bone mass is achieved will help to prevent bone loss as the body ages. The extra calcium in the circulation affects the uptake of calcium into the surface of the bone, reducing bone turnover in the cortical or outer region of the bone. Other effects of the slightly raised calcium level that is present in the blood are that it decreases the level of the circulating parathyroid hormone, which also acts as an inhibitor of bone turnover. Calcium can, therefore, help to prevent bone loss not only in women who have experienced the menopause, but also in those who are suffering bone loss due to the ageing process. In both cases, some loss of bone mass will still occur, but the level of this reduction will depend on the individual.[5,6]

Vitamin D

A number of clinical trials have been undertaken to research the combined use of calcium and vitamin D supplementation. Vitamin D is a major controlling factor in determining how much calcium is absorbed and directed to be taken into the bone. It is now good clinical practice for all patients who are deemed to require treatment for either osteoporosis prevention or the arresting of further bone loss, to be given supplements of calcium and vitamin D. A general health promotion strategy could proceed further, especially in the case of elderly people judged to have a diet containing insufficient quantities of calcium and vitamin D, by providing easily accessible information on ways to increase the level of calcium and vitamin D in the diet. If these dietary improvements cannot be made for some reason, then the persons concerned should be advised to take supplements of these nutrients. Such action should help to hold in abeyance the inevitable onset of loss of bone mass that occurs with age and would prevent elderly people quickly becoming at risk of osteoporosis. More importantly, such measures would reduce the impending threat of any associated fractures, which can considerably affect the individual's quality of life, leading even to death. This type of information could be included in general health promotion literature and be designed in such a way that people would take responsibility for their own health, as they do with similar preventative strategies in coping with other diseases.[7]

The role of calcium and vitamin D in the prevention and treatment of osteoporosis will be discussed in more detail in the following chapter.

Fluoride

Other agents have been used in an attempt to increase calcium uptake into the bone. Chief among these has been fluorine, which is a trace element present in calcified tissue with a particular affinity for bone. Fluoride has been used in the prevention of osteoporosis for a number of years, however clinical studies as to its efficacy have produced rather mixed results. The problem with fluoride is that it has been used in osteoporosis treatment over a long period of time, pre-dating the more modern methods of investigating the efficacy of treatment of osteoporosis. Therefore, in comparison with present-day medications, fluoride has not been subjected to the same rigorous tests, seeking to prove different end points. The level of previous work carried out on fluoride, having no specific merit in further investigations because of the more extensively tested modern drugs, has meant that fluoride has ceased to be a valued treatment.

Fluoride is commonly formulated as the sodium salt, which is freely soluble in aqueous solutions and dissolves easily in the stomach when used in tablet form. The quick and complete dissolution of fluoride tablets means that there is almost 100% absorption, which reaches a peak about 30 minutes after ingestion. The rate and amount of absorption is affected by food, calcium and indigestion mixtures. If a patient is already taking calcium as part of preventative treatment for osteoporosis, then the fluoride must be taken at a different time of day. The use of modified release preparations serves only to help to reduce side-effects and does not alter the amount of fluoride taken up into the skeleton.

The amount of fluoride taken up by the bone is determined by the activity within a specific site of the skeleton: there will be a greater uptake at more active sites rather than at relatively dormant sites. This leads to a selective uptake of fluoride into bone, giving a variation throughout the skeleton and from person to person. This variation may be responsible for the inconsistent results seen in a number of clinical studies.

Fluoride becomes involved in the synthesis of bone by aiding the conversion of amorphous calcium phosphate into octacalcium phosphate and then the hydrolysis of the octacalcium phosphate to hydroxyapatite. This has the overall effect of increasing the synthesis of the hydroxyapatite, a fundamental building block in the production of bone. When fluoride becomes incorporated into the apatite molecule, forming a fluoro-apatite and fluoro-hydroxyapatite, a similar network of apatite molecules is produced, as fluoride is of the same order of size as the hydroxyl group. Unfortunately, this creates a framework that is not as stable as the normal structure, because there are open spaces between the molecules. The benefit is that the fluoride combination molecules are less soluble than the natural apatite molecules, making the fluoride bone more resistant to resorption by the osteoclasts.

The effect of fluoride on the hydroxyapatite crystal is a dose/response-related process, whereby at a low dose or physiological quantity (of the order of 2 mg or less) fluoride acts as a driver in the production of hydroxyapatite. At a therapeutic dose anywhere between 20 mg and 30 mg, the fluoride becomes incorporated into the hydroxyapatite molecule, forming the fluoro derivatives. Further increases in the dose of fluoride, above 30 mg, lead to a large-scale infiltration of the hydroxyapatite crystal, changing its shape and ability to perform within the bone structure.

These changes, attributed to increasing doses of fluoride, can be detected by studying X-rays of the bone because of the distinctive mottling effect apparent on the surface of the bone, together with the presence of osteosclerosis. The use of fluoride is associated with an increase in bone mass, although the method by which this increase is produced is not entirely understood. It is evident that the number of osteoblasts is greater, but they appear to be smaller and possibly have a lower capacity for bone formation. Furthermore, the process of bone formation becomes slower, since the production of the bone matrix takes longer, as does the process of mineralisation. In the presence of high dose fluoride, the consistency of the new bone that is formed changes from the usual lamellar structure into a woven one, which may lead to the development of osteomalacia.

When fluoride is used in combination with calcium, the fluoride acts as a vector, facilitating an increase in the level of the uptake of calcium into the bone; this has the added advantage of either increasing the bone mass or preventing bone loss. The use of vitamin D with fluoride also aids in bone formation and, in combination with calcium, reduces the bone resorption that would occur if either fluoride or vitamin D were used with calcium on their own. However, the use of vitamin D in combination with fluoride, requires to be strictly monitored, because there is a danger of inducing vitamin D toxicity, which would certainly give rise to an increase in bone loss from the cortical bone. Fluoride, when combined with calcium, is seen to have the same effect on bone as the calcium and vitamin D combination.

Fluoride on its own does not affect normal biochemical parameters, but because in most instances fluoride is combined with calcium and vitamin D, any abnormal biochemistry is usually attributed to vitamin D toxicity. These adverse effects of fluoride have a direct result on calcium, manifesting as hypercalcaemia and hypercalciuria arising from the elevated levels of calcium in the circulation. This also causes a secondary hyperparathyroidism when the dietary content of calcium and vitamin D is poor, but can be eliminated if supplements are given.

In order to be effective when given to reduce bone mass loss, fluoride must be administered with calcium and vitamin D supplements. The difficulty arises in attempting to discern exactly which medication is acting as the catalyst, without undertaking a detailed analysis of the bone structure, which is rarely feasible. Thus measuring the various markers of bone metabolism is the only means of determining the possible reasons for the changes in the bone mass. A few radiological studies have indicated some increases in the spinal bone density, in particular an increase in the prominence of trabecular markings and a thickening of the vertebral end plates. Mixed results have been obtained of the effect of fluoride on bone mass. Over a five-year period, dramatic gains in vertebral bone mass have been reported and some evidence of an improvement in the bones of the limbs, but other studies have failed to discover any increase in bone mass in over 40% of the patients treated. Why this should be the case remains unresolved. By contrast, the use of fluoride has failed to produce an increase in the bone mass at cortical bone sites, such as the finger and forearm. In fact, if high doses of fluoride are given in the absence of calcium a decrease in bone width becomes apparent at these cortical bone sites. This condition is probably related to the presence of an increased level of the parathyroid hormone.

The effectiveness of any treatment in osteoporosis is judged by its ability to reduce fractures. This benefit is derived from a combination of improving bone mass and increasing bone strength. Fluoride-treated bone is known to be stronger, but only when measured by compressive forces. The torsional forces created in bone, which may lead to a fracture, either remain unaltered or are reduced with fluoride use.

There is little doubt that fluoride used in conjunction with calcium and vitamin D can help to prevent bone loss and has been reported even to restore bone loss, but there is a great deal of controversy over the benefits, if any, on the prevention of fractures. A number of different dosages and treatment regimens have been tried, but none with consistent results that would indicate the optimum treatment regimen. This outcome could be related more to the study design rather than to the dosage of fluoride, because it has been noted that there was considerable variation in the description of what was termed to be a vertebral fracture in these studies. The only conclusion that can be drawn is that there are many patients who do and many patients who do not respond to fluoride therapy. One other characteristic of fluoride is that it can be formulated in a variety of different salts, leading to discrepancies in the bioavailability, dosage and penetration into bone.

When combined with sufficient quantities of calcium and vitamin D, the one consistent result yielded by fluoride treatment was the relief of the symptoms of back pain shortly after the therapy had commenced. Again, it would be easy to criticise these trials for failing to set the correct parameters or to impose strict controls to ensure the rigor of the results.

The use of any drug produces side-effects and fluoride is no exception. The side-effects of fluoride use are mainly related to irritation of the gastrointestinal tract and range from nausea, vomiting, abdominal pain, diarrhoea through to gastrointestinal bleeding, which is rare. These gastrointestinal side-effects, although common, are usually transient and will diminish with time or can be relieved by the use of an alternative form of the medication, such as an enteric coated or modified-release tablet. One other side-effect caused by fluoride is bone pain, and this is a valid reason for discontinuing treatment because it has been found that once fluoride has been withdrawn, the pain is often eliminated within 4–8 weeks of stopping the therapy. In some instances, the bone pain is associated with microfractures or fissure fractures occurring after bone calluses have formed, but seldom is the bone pain associated with a complete fracture. The incidence of bone pain is more often experienced by patients with a low BMD, and in such cases the fluoride should be withdrawn either until the pain is resolved or the cause of the pain is isolated and treated. If microfractures are the root cause of the bone pain, then once these fractures are eliminated, the fluoride can be reintroduced at a lower dose in order to prevent further pain and the possible recurrence of the microfractures.

In some clinical trials the use of fluoride has led to reports of an increase in the incidence of hip fractures within the treatment group, but these reports have been inconsistent. After analysing a number of different clinical studies that employed various treatment schedules, the evidence would appear to suggest that there was no change in the hip fracture rate, and that a reduction in the number of hip fractures was evident when fluoride was combined with calcium and vitamin D.

In conclusion, the administration of fluoride proves beneficial to those patients showing the signs and symptoms of the early stages of osteoporosis, but would be best avoided in patients with marked cortical osteoporosis in order to avoid the risk of bone pain and of possible hip fractures. In adults, fluoride has been given in doses of up to 30 mg per day, but if adverse gastrointestinal effects arise consideration should be given either to reducing the dose or to changing the formulation of the tablet, to one that is enteric coated or of modified release. The success of the therapy would require to be monitored by carrying out BMD measurements on a regular basis. Since most of the patients are likely to be elderly, they will probably be suffering from impaired renal function, which must be taken into consideration prior to commencing the treatment. Fluoride should be given with calcium supplements to enhance the benefits and limit the side-effects. Vitamin D supplements should be prescribed only when the patient is lacking in this vitamin or when dietary sources are insufficient. In order to ensure a reasonable prospect of success in preventing osteoporosis progression, the treatment should extend over a five-year period. If the fluoride is discontinued earlier, bone loss will gradually revert, over a number of years, to the pretreatment level. Treatment could be safely given over a further five-year span, providing the medication is tolerated and depending on the effect on the bone loss.

The use of fluoride as a preventative treatment for osteoporosis has largely been superseded by the use of other drugs, which have achieved more successful clinical results in a number of trials.[2,8]

Hormone replacement therapy

The next breakthrough occurred when it was discovered that women who had been prescribed hormone replacement therapy (HRT) for treatment of postmenopausal symptoms maintained a slower rate of bone loss for as long as the treatment continued in comparison with those women who were not receiving any treatment. The use, of HRT is now the mainstay of preventative therapy for osteoporosis in post-menopausal women. This group of drugs is presently available in a wide variety of dosage forms in order to aid compliance and to reduce the number and the severity of side-effects. The recent addition of selective oestrogen receptor modulators offers a further option that is reputed to have a cleaner side-effect profile, in particular for those women at risk of breast cancer.[3]

This use of HRT is discussed in more detail in Chapter 9.

Bisphosphonates

The bisphosphonates are currently prescribed to prevent osteoporosis in patients who have been taking systemic corticosteroids on a long-term basis and at doses in excess of the physiological level. In these cases, the bisphosphonates assist by preventing bone suppression caused by the use of the corticosteroids. Furthermore, because no equivalent to female HRT exists for the prevention of osteoporosis in men, bisphosphonates remain the sole form of drug therapy that is recommended for men. They are discussed in more detail in Chapter 10.

Active treatment

Active treatment for osteoporosis consists of the initiation of drug therapy to actively increase bone mass when there is the need to prevent either an initial fracture or the likelihood of sustaining a second fracture. In such patients there will have been a definitive diagnosis of osteo-porosis following a critical incident, such as a low-impact fracture, or after a confirming bone density measurement using a diagnostic test, for example a DEXA scanner.

Anabolic steroids

The role of anabolic steroids in maintaining various bodily functions or enhancing these functions in order to improve efficiency in the human body has been known for many years. It is because of this knowledge that anabolic steroids have been used as an aid to improve body metabolism and to act as a pick-me-up or tonic. Although medically this use can no longer be approved because the adverse longer term effects far outweigh the benefits, certain athletes have persisted in the misuse of anabolic steroids in order to improve their body condition. On the other hand, it is because of certain therapeutic effects of particular anabolic steroids that these have been proposed as an active treatment to combat osteoporosis.

The therapeutic role of anabolic steroids in the treatment of osteoporosis has been known for over 50 years. These steroids create an advantageous calcium balance in the skeleton. The first steroid to be used in this way was testosterone, either on its own or in combination with oestrogen. The one major drawback with this therapy, which made it unacceptable to women, who were the majority of the patients being treated, is that it has masculinisation side-effects.

In an attempt to overcome these side-effects a number of derivatives of testosterone have been proposed; but although these drugs have less androgenic effects and there has been a reduction in the masculinisation in comparison with testosterone, the adverse effects have not been eliminated and are dose-dependent.

There are two main types of anabolic steroids based on their chemical structure around the carbon 17 position within the steroid molecule. These structural differences in the molecule separate the oral preparations of stanozolol and oxymethalone from the injectable forms of testosterone and nandrolone.

The anabolic steroids cause a significant reduction in the amount of calcium excreted. This is related to the reduction of calcium released from bone, because the anabolic steroids affect both bone formation and bone resorption. It is not clear whether the anabolic steroids exclusively stimulate bone formation or reduce bone resorption or affect both functions in a way that creates a net bone mass increase. The specific mechanism of action has not yet been elucidated since, during treatment with anabolic steroids, the level of the usual biochemical bone markers does not change from the normal range.

The reduction in the calcium level in the urine is thought to be from a direct effect of the steroid on the parathyroid hormone. The reason for this is that the calcium blood level is unaffected as there is an increase in renal reabsorption of calcium. This suggests that the effect of the parathyroid hormone on the renal tubular system is enhanced due to an increase in its potency on the kidney caused by the anabolic steroid.

As previously stated, the mechanism of action of the anabolic steroids is not fully understood, but it is known that during treatment the number and activity of osteoblasts are raised. The anabolic steroid stimulates the osteoblasts, leading to an increase in bone formation in developing bone. This increase in bone formation is countered by an increase in the level of osteoclasts, which produce more bone erosions as a source of bone resorption. These observations give rise to the belief that certain anabolic steroids, namely stanozolol and nandrolone, increase the total activity of bone remodelling.

The net effect of this increase in activity is that the bone mass increases at cortical bone sites. This is seen not only in the first year, but continues into the second year at the same rate, and can be explained by the rise in total body calcium. It is not known whether the changes in bone mass continue in subsequent years after the second year or if at some point a steady state is reached. Longer duration studies would need to be carried out to establish this.

The increase in bone mass must be put into context, as anabolic steroids also change the body composition, causing a decrease in the ratio of fat to muscle. This change will affect the ability of various diagnostic tests to measure the bone density as accurately as prior to treatment, and this could lead to higher than expected levels of bone density caused by the change in soft tissue surrounding the bone. Even after the cessation of treatment with the anabolic steroid, the bone mass remains roughly the same, despite the rapid reversal of the body fat metabolism and thus content that occurs over a few months.

Unfortunately, this evidence of increase in bone mass is not substantiated by significant data on the reduction of fractures. The perception is that the relative risk of both vertebrae and hip fractures is reduced, but there are no hard data to confirm this. Evidence to support this theory is that the anabolic steroids improve the level of muscle compared with a reduction in body fat, which increases muscular power and helps to improve not only the patient's mobility but the patient's confidence in his or her ability to cope with the activities of daily life. Thus it could be that the overall benefit of anabolic steroids in the prevention of fractures is the reduction of the possibility of patients suffering a low-impact fracture by having either the ability to avoid these situations or the capacity to endure the injury without sustaining a fracture.

The side-effect profile of anabolic steroids is well known, from both misuse by athletes, such as weight lifters, and from therapeutic use. The main side-effect is liver toxicity, which is usually identified as an elevation of liver enzymes, up to twice the normal upper level. These liver effects are coupled with an alteration of the lipid profile, increasing the risk of atheroma in the cardiovascular system. These side-effects must be weighed against the benefits prior to the commencement of the treatment and monitored during the treatment, since these effects would be a reason for discontinuation. Other side-effects, which the female patient ought to be aware of, include the manifestation of male characteristics, in particular, hoarseness of voice and other body changes. The choice of drug and the dosage regimen can be altered to limit these adverse effects. Some of these drugs will cause an irreversible change in the voice, which limits the length of time the treatment can be given.

Sodium and water retention can also be troublesome side-effects. These can be treated with diuretics if they persist, but they do not normally constitute a reason for stopping the treatment.

The presence of the above side-effects has curtailed the therapeutic use of anabolic steroids. Even with the expected benefits obtained in previous clinical trials, treatment regimens are rarely able to mimic the duration of treatment required and therefore very little benefit was obtained. This has led to the limiting of their clinical use to elderly patients, who would benefit from the bone and muscle improvements; over and above this, there have been the anecdotal reports of confidence boosting. Even restriction of treatment to the elderly has been questioned, leading to anabolic steroids failing to be recommended to these patients. Furthermore, with the advent of alternative safer treatments the use of anabolic steroids has been all but superseded.[2,9]

Testosterone

In men with osteoporosis, treatment with testosterone has usually been reserved for patients lacking in the production of testosterone. Hence, the testosterone is given as a hormone replacement therapy in order to restore levels to a normal range and to have an effect on restoring bone mass. Even men who have a normal level of testosterone can benefit from replacement therapy, as this has been shown to produce a small increase in bone mass. This result has only been reported in short-term studies.

The difficulty with the use of testosterone is that it is not easily available as an oral or intramuscular preparation; the testosterone has to be formulated as a long-acting ester of the hormone to prevent rapid metabolism and a short duration of action. Until recently, the only form of testosterone for long-term therapy was the intramuscular depot injection, but with the introduction of the transdermal patch and an oral capsule patients do have other options.

Bisphosphonates

The only drug treatment that is used as active therapy not only for reversing bone loss but also to actively promote bone resorption are the bisphosphonates. Normally bisphosphonates are only initiated once a positive diagnosis of osteoporosis has been made. If preventative treatment has already been started but has failed to prevent further signs or symptoms of osteoporosis, combination therapy may be employed to reverse the continuous degeneration of bone.

The bisphosphonates are often used in combination with calcium and vitamin D supplementation, as this is seen as a synergistic treatment with one augmenting the other, leading to a greater response than would be expected if each drug were to be used separately.

Bisphosphonates are the one therapy that can be used as either prevention or treatment, depending on the stage of the disease. Bisphosphonates are the only treatment that can be identified as increasing bone mass, in comparison with the other previously mentioned drugs, which merely decelerate the progressive bone loss that occurs with age.

The bisphosphonates have now superseded other drugs, such as fluoride and anabolic steroids, in the active treatment of osteoporosis. Since these drugs were introduced they have been formulated to aid compliance, initially as a once-a-day continuous therapy, then as a once-a-week treatment and finally being developed into an injection to be given monthly to yearly. Bisphosphonates offer the greatest promise for the treatment of osteoporosis at the moment, although they all pose a problem with regard to upper gastrointestinal side-effects.

Other therapies

Osteoporosis will develop in a patient with underlying hypothyroidism if this condition is left untreated. Therefore, levothyroxine, if given in supplementary doses, will prevent and reverse the development of osteoporosis. The dose requires to be monitored closely to achieve a therapeutic response, as both hyperthyroidism and hypothyroidism will lead to osteoporosis.

The administration of supplementary calcitonin, a hormone secreted by the parathyroid gland and a potent inhibitor of osteoclasts, will affect bone resorption, leading to a reduction in bone loss. Calcitonin is normally given as the salmon derivative called salcatonin in the form of a subcutaneous injection. The inconvenience of continually giving a subcutaneous injection and the high acquisition cost has led to this therapy largely being ignored.

One group of drugs that is commonly used in the treatment of the elderly for other indications, but which also has a beneficial effect on osteoporosis, is the thiazide diuretics, which are indicated for hypertension and heart failure. The thiazide diuretics cause an increase in tubular reabsorption of calcium, which has the effect of increasing serum calcium, decreasing parathyroid hormone, reducing intestinal calcium absorption and bone turnover.

However, although the thiazides have been advocated for use in osteoporosis, there has been no large prospective clinical trial to prove their efficacy either in increasing bone mass or in reducing fracture rate. A number of studies have indicated that patients taking thiazides for hypertension have shown an increase in bone mineral density in comparison with patients who have been given other treatments for hypertension.[10]

References

1. Royal College of Physicians. *Osteoporosis. Clinical Guidelines for Prevention and Treatment*. London: Royal College of Physicians, 1999.
2. Kanis J A. *Osteoporosis*. Oxford: Blackwell Science, 1996.
3. Prevention and treatment of osteoporosis. *MeReC Bull* 1999; **10**: 25–28.
4. Drugs for prevention and treatment of osteoporosis. *Medical Letter* 2000; **42**: 97–100.
5. The North American Menopause Society (consensus opinion). *Menopause* 2001; **8**: 84–95.
6. Mason P. Calcium – an update. *Pharm J* 2002; **268**: 329–330.
7. Chapuy M C, Arlot M E, Duboeuf F, *et al.* Vitamin D and calcium to prevent hip fractures in elderly women. *N Engl J Med* 1992; **327**: 1637–1642.
8. Reginster J Y, Meurmans L, Zegels B, *et al.* The effect of sodium monofluorophosphate plus calcium on vertebral fracture rate in postmenopausal women with moderate osteoporosis: a randomised controlled trial. *Ann Intern Med* 1998; **129**: 1–8.
9. *British National Formulary* No. 46. London: British Medical Association and Royal Pharmaceutical Society, 2003.
10. Rubin M R, Bilezikian J P. New anabolic therapies in osteoporosis. *Curr Opin Rheumatol* 2002; **14**: 433–440.

8

Calcium and vitamin D

Osteoporosis is looked upon as a disease of the elderly, but the seeds of this condition are sown throughout life. In previous chapters the role of various lifestyle factors has been explained, including the importance of the diet. It is well known that calcium and vitamin D are required for the development of strong bones and teeth during the formative years. The lack of these nutrients produces a deficiency disease, which is recognised by deformities of the body, in particular of the long bones. The reduction in the incidence of this deficiency disease has been brought about by ensuring that the general population receives enough calcium and vitamin D in their diet. On the whole, people in the Western world are living longer because of the improvement in overall health due to better public healthcare and the awareness of the benefits of a healthy lifestyle. All these changes have thrown up a new set of problems, one of which is the increasing incidence of osteoporosis in the ageing population. This has increased the knowledge of the value of the building blocks of bone tissue, how it is maintained and how to prevent the gradual loss of bone with age. Therefore, it is only natural to identify the constituents of bone and discover the ways in which to influence the fundamental processes for a beneficial outcome in osteoporosis. This is why, at this stage, a thorough examination of the role played by calcium and vitamin D is necessary in order to evaluate the evidence for treatment and prevention. The two nutrients are discussed together because they are both involved in the mechanism for the homeostasis of the skeleton.[1]

Calcium

There is a common misconception that the skeleton is a rigid, non-living structure and that once bones achieve their maximum growth there is no further development and, to all intents and purposes, the bones are dead tissue.

Nothing could be further from the truth; bone tissue is a dynamic system at a cellular level, and there is a continual breakdown and reformation of bone. The bone can be thought of as a production line, along which tissue is being constantly renewed through turnover, metabolism and remodelling.

In order to maintain this activity within bone there is a requirement to ensure that all the building blocks, in the form of nutrients, are present in sufficient quantities. This consideration is at the root of the use of calcium in the initial stages of prevention and, to some extent, treatment of osteoporosis. The basis of this approach is founded on the fact that bones possess a high calcium content; therefore, by giving the patient large doses of calcium the bone can continue to remodel itself without being checked due to lack of raw material.

The calcium content of bone reaches a peak in the early part of adult life, after which there is a slow but gradual decline in bone mass and thus a release of calcium from the bone. In men, this decline continues throughout life at roughly the same pace, until later life, when there is a slight acceleration, usually in the seventh and eighth decade. In women, the peak bone mass is slightly lower, but the rate of loss of bone mass is similar to that in men until the menopause, when it increases sharply. The menopause is a major pivotal event in bone development. During this period there is a rapid loss of bone mass together with a loss of calcium over a relatively short period. Once the menopause is complete, however, the bone loss rate returns to the level in existence before the menopause, and as time goes on the loss may become even slower due to the much-reduced bone content.

There are a number of factors that will facilitate the prediction of an individual's possible peak bone mass. As seen in earlier chapters, this is greatly influenced by what was inherited and to a lesser extent by diet, exercise and other lifestyle factors. It is known that if a person is deficient in calcium and vitamin D whilst growing up, then rickets, a deficiency disease, may develop. This deficiency disease leads to the production of bones that are weak and soft, giving rise to malformation of the bones, in particular of the weight-bearing bones. This knowledge supports the widespread prescribing of calcium to patients who are known to be suffering from osteoporosis, but as is seen with the deficiency disease rickets, this is not the whole story.

A number of studies have been carried out into the use of calcium supplements in the prevention of osteoporosis. Initially, this mineral was given in doses similar to those used in the treatment of deficiency diseases, but evidence has shown that larger doses are required, with anything from 600 mg (15 mmol) to 1.5 g (37.5 mmol) of elemental calcium per day being given as a supplement. This is in addition to the calcium content of the diet, which on average, is in the region of 600 mg per day. Mixed results have been obtained, ranging from claims that 'the use of supplements has made no difference over placebo'[2] to others that 'the use of supplements has led to the prevention of crush vertebral fractures'.[3] In order to clarify the role of calcium in osteoporosis there is a need to look in greater depth at what happens when calcium is taken into the skeleton.[4]

The role of calcium in bone

Bone contains of a number of defined units called bone modelling units or basic multicellular units (BMU), which are continually undergoing a cycle of remodelling. This remodelling process within trabecular bone commences with activation, then resorption by osteoclasts and finally bone formation, and each BMU evolves through the stages of remodelling at its own rate. The number of BMUs present in a section of bone will define the bone volume, formation and resorption rate: the smaller the number of BMUs, the lower the rate of bone formation and resorption. During bone remodelling, each BMU resorbs more bone than it forms; this is why, in the adult, there is a gradual loss of bone mass. If bone remodelling could be halted by inhibiting the activation phase, but yet allowing the bone formation to continue, then bone volume would increase by about 5–10%, depending on the initial rate of bone remodelling. The full effects would not be apparent for about three months, which equates to one bone formation period. The bone would then continue to stabilise at this increased volume.

It is thought that calcium, when taken in doses in excess of the body's replacement requirements, acts as a biofeedback mechanism on the parathyroid hormone thus reducing its release. This partial inhibition of the parathyroid hormone release has a direct effect on the activation phase of the bone remodelling process. Although there is a decrease in bone activation, this is not sufficient to create a marked improvement in bone formation; however it may reduce the rate of bone loss. In the presence of calcium deficiency, supplementation will bring about an increase in bone mass due to the improvement in mineralisation of the existing bone.[5]

Calcium absorption

The absorption of calcium, like many other dietary nutrients, takes place through the mucosa of the small intestine, which is the major site of absorption from the intestine. In general, the average diet consists of about 25 mmol calcium (1 g of elemental calcium); of which around 10 mmol (400 mg) is absorbed, with approximately 5 mmol (200 mg) being actively secreted by the intestine, directly or via the bile and pancreatic secretions. In conclusion, the outcome of this process, results in only 5 mmol (200 mg) entering the extracellular fluid and being available for use by the body.

The availability of calcium from the diet also depends on the nature of the food source, because the presence of certain salts such as phosphates, oxalates and phytates will inhibit absorption. These salts combine with calcium to produce either insoluble compounds or calcium that is bound to insoluble organic matter. This reduces the potential of calcium to be absorbed and is an initial constraint on the amount of calcium available. Therefore, when the dietary calcium is mainly derived from dairy products it is more easily absorbed due to the presence of soluble salts than when it is obtained from vegetables, which contain mainly phytates and oxalates.

There are two mechanisms of absorption of calcium from the gastrointestinal tract: active transport under the influence of vitamin D carried out in the duodenum and upper part of the jejunum, and diffusion, which occurs in the rest of the gastrointestinal tract, distal to the duodenum. Although active transport is normally a major contributor to absorption, in the case of calcium the number of sites is relatively small compared to the large area of intestine available for diffusion so the contrary is true.

Calcium absorption is under the control of the parathyroid hormone, calcitonin and the various vitamin D metabolites: these substances maintain the level of calcium within the extracellular fluid. If the body needs to increase or decrease the serum calcium level, it will actively secrete parathyroid hormone and calcitonin, which will increase both the efficiency of calcium absorption and the transfer into the bone. If vitamin D levels are reduced, due to either deficiency or malabsorption, this will reduce calcium absorption by curtailing the active transport mechanism.

These processes are sufficient to deal with any short-term variations in the availability of calcium from the diet. In the longer term, due to chronic changes in requirements or in dietary content, intervention with supplements will be necessary.[5]

Calcium supplements

Traditionally, the use of calcium supplements have been recommended for the treatment of deficiency states and the content of the available

MANAGEMENT FOCUS

Calcium and vitamin D dosages per day
Calcium 1 g (elemental)
Vitamin D 20 µg (800 units)

products has been tailored for that purpose. Until recently, calcium supplements contained between 1 and 2 mmol (40–80 mg) calcium in a chewable or soluble formulation, given at least twice a day. It is now recognised that this dose is totally inadequate. The minimum dose advised is now 1 g of elemental calcium (25 mmol) (see Management Focus, above). Often doses in excess of this are used, up to and including 50 mmol (2 g). Formulations are generally in soluble or chewable forms, which are designed to be palatable and easy to take. The soluble preparations ensure that the calcium is taken with plenty of water, not only to facilitate ingestion but also to help with absorption. There is little difference in taking the calcium with food or without food, as this does not significantly affect the absorption of the calcium from the supplement. Similarly the splitting of the dose into two divided doses will increase absorption but this will not affect overall clinical outcome.

Calcium salts, which are used in the various preparations, differ in the content of elemental calcium. This is an important consideration, as the salt can constitute anything from 60% to 90% of the content by weight. Calcium carbonate is commonly used, as it can be formulated into a soluble and chewable form; furthermore, it contains the largest content of calcium by weight (40%). The bioavailabilty of the calcium varies depending on the salt chosen. There is evidence available to support the claim that the citrate salt produces the most efficient absorption; but this is only significant in patients with achlorhydria.

It is important for patients at risk of osteoporosis or with the established disease to take calcium as a supplement over several years if the benefits of the therapy are to be maintained. This means that the patient needs to be willing to take the calcium every day, which may be difficult if the calcium preparation offered is unpalatable. In recent years, this problem has been recognised by the pharmaceutical manufacturers, and various once-daily calcium supplements that are formulated into flavoured drinks or tablets or granules that melt in the mouth have been developed. These improved formulations have greatly enhanced patient concordance because the calcium is no longer looked upon as a twice per day penance, in the shape of tablets which tasted like chalk, no matter how they were disguised or with what they were combined.[6]

Calcium and bone density

The use of calcium supplements at more than physiological doses has been shown to reduce the rate of bone loss in the absence of any other treatment. This is particularly marked when the dose of calcium is of the order of 1 g of elemental calcium per day. In the case of the bone loss from the cortical bone in postmenopausal women, such doses may halve the rate of loss. This beneficial effect on cortical bone and especially on trabecular bone in women is prolonged well into later life. The use of calcium in postmenopausal women is seen to reduce bone loss considerably, to the extent that the actual bone loss is practically negligible in comparison with the 1% loss that occurs in women who have not taken the calcium supplement. In some long-term studies, this effective use of calcium has been noted to continue for a period of up to four years. In postmenopausal women, if calcium supplementation is combined with an exercise programme, then this has a marked effect on bone mineral density, especially when the dose of calcium is of the order of 1 g per day.

This reduction in bone loss caused by calcium supplementation can be explained by its effect in reducing bone turnover, which is probably caused by the small elevation of serum calcium level inhibiting the secretion of the parathyroid hormone. The resultant reduction in activation of bone turnover would account for the increase in skeletal mass that is often seen in individuals taking calcium supplements.

Calcium supplementation is often combined with vitamin D, which increases calcium absorption from the gastrointestinal tract, thus improving the possibility of increasing bone mass and preventing bone loss. Other beneficial effects are seen when calcium is combined with an anti-resorptive agent, such as hormone replacement therapy, either as oestrogen or as the combined product with a progestogen. In a similar manner, calcium combined with additional active treatments, namely calcitonin, has shown the same synergistic effects in comparison with monotherapy.

The addition of calcium to other active treatments in osteoporosis has prompted the majority of the clinical trials with the newer drugs, such as the bisphosphonates, to incorporate calcium as part of the standard therapy. Thus, in comparative trials both the control arm of the study and those taking the placebo are given calcium, which is seen as the minimum therapy for osteoporotic patients.

If calcium is given to a patient taking a thiazide diuretic, then the calcium level in the blood will be raised by the action of the thiazide on the kidney, which increases the reabsorption of the calcium. This not only increases the amount of available calcium, but also increases uptake into bone. Although this is clearly of benefit in osteoporosis, particularly if calcium is not well tolerated, it will need to be closely monitored in case of hypercalcaemia.[7]

Calcium and fracture rate

Although calcium supplementation can be seen to increase overall skeletal mass and decrease bone turnover, evidence of a reduction in fracture rate of either vertebrae or hip is limited. In comparative clinical trials, calcium supplementation often does have an effect when compared with placebo, but the difference is rarely significant. This could be accounted for by the fact that a number of years of taking calcium are necessary before any results are noticeable, while on the other hand any gain is rapidly lost on cessation of the treatment. If the clinical trial is conducted over a relatively short period, such as one or two years, then the full therapeutic effect of calcium will not be seen.

In population studies that have looked at the dietary intake of calcium amongst women, those who had a higher intake of calcium had a reduced fracture rate. However, this reduction in fracture rate could not be solely identified as resulting from the high dietary calcium because there were other differences between the two groups. In particular, the women with a high-calcium diet were more motivated through education and knowledge of health in general.[5]

In one study that examined the use of calcium supplements in perimenopausal women, it was shown that over a two-year period of supplementation there was a reduction in vertebral bone loss. There was also a significant increase in urinary calcium, whereas there was a decrease in the urinary excretion of various biochemical markers. The bone loss was less marked in the second year than in the first, which suggests a stabilisation of bone loss and bone turnover.[8]

Side-effects

When taken by mouth, calcium supplementation at doses of 1 or 2 mmol will have few, if any, side-effects. At the larger doses required for the treatment of osteoporosis, mild gastrointestinal side-effects are often seen, such as bloating or constipation due to decreased gut motility.[9]

Vitamin D

There are two sources of vitamin D: through the action of sunlight on the skin and through the diet. The main source is through synthesis in the skin from the action of ultraviolet light on 7-dehydrocholesterol, a precursor sterol. There is sufficient vitamin D produced from this process during the months of sunlight to build up stores within the body to survive the sunlight-depleted months in temperate climes. However, if sunlight exposure is restricted for whatever reason, then adequate stores of vitamin D will not be generated and deficiency diseases, such as osteomalacia, may develop. This sometimes occurs in elderly people, who tend to spend more time indoors than the rest of the population. It can also be compounded in northern countries by the reduced level of sunlight, but even in southern European cities sunlight has difficulty in penetrating between tall buildings in towns and cities. The custom of wearing black clothing by elderly women in some Mediterranean cultures decreases the sun's ability to manufacture vitamin D, while in other cultures elderly women are at risk of vitamin D deficiency if they are restricted to living entirely within the home.

Vitamin D from the diet does not play such an important role, because the quantity of vitamin D is relatively small compared with that derived from ultraviolet light synthesis. It is necessary that vitamin D is derived from both sources in order to maintain the body's stores, especially over the winter months. Foods containing vitamin D include fish liver oils, dairy products and fortified foods, for example margarine. In countries where vegetable oils are used predominantly for cooking this can lead to a lack of vitamin D in the diet, since these oils contain no vitamin D.[10]

Physiology

Vitamin D is necessary for the regulation of absorption of both phosphate and calcium; it achieves this by increasing the absorption from the gastrointestinal tract. Furthermore, it promotes the resorption of calcium from bone, taking forward the process of bone mineralisation whilst maintaining the plasma levels of calcium and phosphate.

The source of vitamin D will determine the structural form of the molecule produced. Colecalciferol (vitamin D_3) is formed as a result of the action of ultraviolet light on 7-dehydrocholesterol in the skin of animals, whereas ergocalciferol (vitamin D_2) is derived synthetically from the irradiation of a plant sterol. Both forms of vitamin D are active in humans and can be used in metabolic pathways to produce the available form responsible for the actions of vitamin D.

Once vitamin D is absorbed into the plasma it has first to undergo hydroxylation within the liver to form 25-hydroxyvitamin D. There is a second hydroxylation in the kidney to produce 1,25-dihydroxyvitamin D (calcitriol); this is the active form of the vitamin. Without these two hydroxylations, the vitamin D will not be effective; therefore, if there is any disruption of these enzymatic processes due to either liver or kidney failure, the vitamin D available will have a reduced function.

Vitamin D and its various hydroxylated forms are transported to the liver and the kidney via a circulating carrier protein. This carrier protein also transports the active form of vitamin D to the target organs, namely the intestine and the skeleton, where it is responsible for calcium regulation. Its major role is at the intestinal site, where calcium supply is maintained. In the skeleton, the active vitamin D is stored, to be used later to stimulate bone resorption and inhibit collagen synthesis, probably in conjunction with parathyroid hormone.

In the absence of vitamin D, the process of bone mineralisation is impaired, leading to the lack of calcification in osteoid tissue. This can be corrected by giving supplements. Why vitamin D deficiency leads to impairment of bone mineralisation has not been clearly defined, but it is thought to be due to a combination of lack of vitamin D metabolites and calcium caused by malabsorption. Further regulation of bone activity is carried out by the 1-α-hydroxylase enzyme present in the kidney, which controls the conversion of vitamin D to its active form, 1,25-dihydroxyvitamin D. This enables the bones to adapt during periods of high demand, such as growth, pregnancy and lactation, so that levels of vitamin D are maintained, despite there being no apparent increase in the availability.[5]

Skeletal effects

The level of vitamin D has direct effects on both the physiology and the structure of bone. Physiologically, the osteoblasts present on the surface of the bone have vitamin D receptors, which on occupation by vitamin D, lead to the production of osteocalcin (bone Gla protein). Once these metabolic steps are complete the resultant osteoblast undergoes further transformation, which is all part of the process of bone mineralisation. This involves the calcification of the osteoblast cell, followed by elongation and, eventually, flattening, before incorporation into the structure of the bone.

The frequency and the rate of the mineralisation depends on the amount of vitamin D in circulation as this affects the number of receptors on the surface osteoblasts. This in turn controls the production of osteocalcin, the level of which is a determining factor in the absorption of minerals onto the bone matrix. In the absence of vitamin D it can be seen that the lack of mineralisation will reduce the production of new bone, leading to an undermining of the strength of the existing bone.[5]

Clinical studies

Vitamin D in combination with calcium has been used in a number of clinical trials in order to investigate its efficacy in increasing the bone mass and reducing fracture rates in postmenopausal women and elderly men. The use of vitamin D with calcium in this way seems to produce greater benefit than either of the two supplements on its own. The reasons for this have not been identified.

It has been shown that a dose of 20 µg (800 units) of vitamin D, given as a divided dose, in combination with calcium can significantly reduce the incidence of hip fractures in an elderly population, some with pre-existing deficiency disease. Such evidence supports the premise that the use of these supplements can still have definitive action late in life, when bone loss is marked and the risk of fracture is high.

This implies that the potential for benefit is not limited solely to those 'becoming at risk', and that, if anything, those at greater risk in later life will profit more from the use of these supplements in the lessening of the occurrence of fractures. Calcium and vitamin D used in conjunction provide a cost-effective therapeutic intervention in the prevention of osteoporotic fractures.

The use of vitamin D has also been shown to have a beneficial effect on muscle strength, and in so doing gives better support to the adjacent bone. This is of particular benefit where there has been a degree of wasting of the muscle, which can occur with age. The improvement in muscle strength can act as an aid to the prevention of falls by both promoting better balance and the ability to sustain or reduce the force of a fall.[11]

Alfacalcidol (1α-Hydroxycholecalciferol)

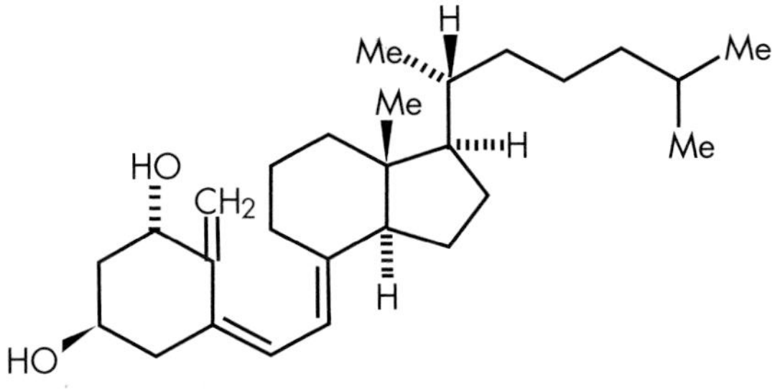

1,25-dihydroxyvitamin D (calcitriol)

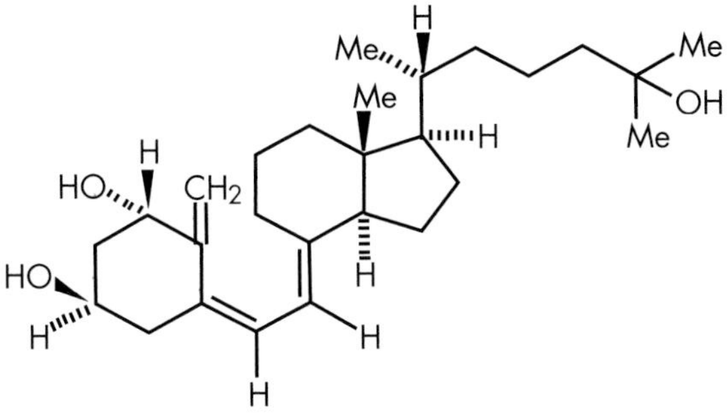

Ergocalciferol (vitamin D$_2$)

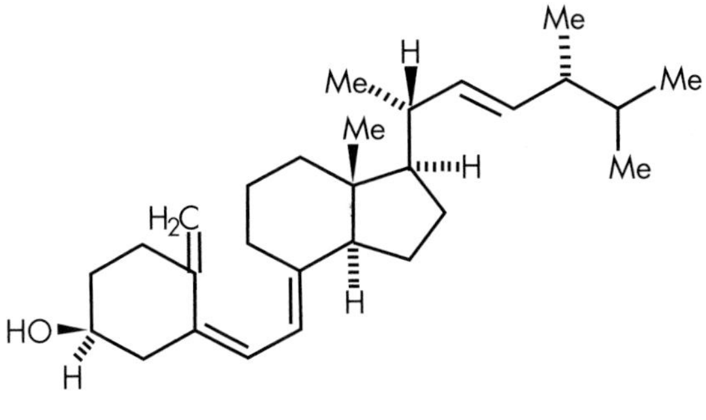

Figure 8.1   Three vitamin D analogues used in the treatment of osteoporosis.

Vitamin D analogues: calcitriol, alfacalcidol and ergocalciferol

The use of these derivatives of vitamin D (see Figure 8.1) has been mainly restricted to the adjuvant treatment of kidney and liver disease, where there is a lack of the converting enzyme that activates the

MANAGEMENT FOCUS

Vitamin D and its analogues used in the treatment of osteoporosis
Vitamin D_2 – Ergocalciferol – requires hydroxylation in the kidney and liver for activation.
Alfacalcidol – 1α-Hydroxycholecalciferol – used in renal disease supplementation.
Calcitriol – 1,25-Dihydroxycholecalciferol – used in liver disease supplementation.

absorbed vitamin D. Alfacalcidol needs to undergo hydroxylation in the liver before it is transformed into the active form of vitamin D, calcitriol.

These analogues of vitamin D increase calcium absorption from the small intestine, leading to an increase in osteocalcin and a decrease in the parathyroid hormone. Calcium serum and urinary levels are increased because of the increase in the absorption of calcium, with a reduction in the bone remodelling.

The effect of this increase in calcium has the direct result of increasing bone mass; this can be by as much as 10–20% of the skeletal mass. Any benefit derived from this appears to be dependent on the calcium and nutritional status of the individual. Where there is the greatest need that is where the greatest improvement will show. In a number of studies the results have ranged from 'no change at all' to 'great improvement', although not sustained. Possible reasons for these variations in response are that calcitriol has a narrow therapeutic window, which would limit the response to a standard dosage regimen (see Management Focus, above).[5]

Fracture results

A number of studies have carried out research into the use of both calcitriol and alfacalcidol and their ability to reduce vertebral fractures. These are at best variable, differences stemming from the designs of the studies and the use of combinations with other therapeutic modalities. For instance, although good results are obtained with alfacalcidol, these responses were from the larger trials, which were all open trials in which alfacalcidol was used either on its own or combined with variable amounts of calcium or as in one case with a form of calcitonin. Although all the clinical trials showed a consistent reduction in vertebral fractures, the variation in design leads to a lack of reproducibility of both the results and the side-effects reported.

The results of clinical trials of calcitriol are more disappointing because there were a number of negative trials. This could be accounted for by the fact that the trials were not sensitive enough to identify the full clinical effect of calcitriol. One clinical trial that did show beneficial effects, was a three-year trial comparing calcitriol with calcium. In this study the reduction in vertebral fractures became apparent only in the second and third years of the trial.[12]

Side-effects

The major problem occurring in the use of both of these analogues of vitamin D is the incidence and degree of hypercalcaemia. It is therefore critical that the amount of calcium both in the diet and in any supplements given is closely monitored. Furthermore, frequent measurements of serum calcium levels are important in the early stages of treatment to prevent hypercalcaemia. The use of these analogues brings about a fast response, which allows for a quick titration of dose; but if overlooked, the rise in calcium may lead to prolonged hypercalcaemia, kidney damage and nephrocalcinosis.

Formulations

Until recently, the only method by which vitamin D could be given on a regular basis as an oral preparation was in combination with calcium in tablet form. When two of these tablets were administered they contained sufficient vitamin D, but the level of calcium included was a tenth of that required in osteoporosis. Now that research has established the correct dose of calcium and vitamin D for the prevention and treatment of osteoporosis, reliance on an underdosing combination preparation is no longer necessary. A number of pharmaceutical manufacturers have realised the need for a high-dose calcium and vitamin D preparation for osteoporosis. Patients now have to take only one or two of the same tablet per day in order to obtain the necessary dose of calcium and vitamin D, rather than having to swallow a combination of different tablets in order to achieve the required dose.[9]

Combination therapy

It is well recognised that in the prevention and treatment of osteoporosis, supplementation with calcium and vitamin D should be in place before other therapies are considered. Calcium and vitamin D are now commonly given as part of treatment regimen for osteoporosis with other therapies in order to ensure that these basic nutrients are available to promote the desired increase in bone mass. Any major clinical research into osteoporosis requires that when a new drug is compared with controls, both arms of the study have adequate calcium and vitamin D.

Drug interactions

Although calcium and vitamin D are readily available from the diet, they do have the potential to interact with several drug therapies. More to the point, they will readily combine with other treatments used in the prevention and treatment of osteoporosis.

Calcium often combines with salts of drugs to produce insoluble products; examples of these are the tetracyclines and ciprofloxacin. This type of interaction is evident in its use with bisphosphonates, which will combine with calcium if taken together, limiting absorption of both calcium and the bisphosphonate. To prevent this happening, the two medications should be taken at least two hours apart, which is enough time to allow one drug to be absorbed before the second is taken. The usual advice is to take the bisphosphonate first thing in the morning, at least two hours prior to eating breakfast; the calcium can then be taken with or after breakfast.[9]

There is also a drug interaction between thiazide diuretics and calcium, leading to excessive calcium in the body since thiazides conserve calcium in the kidney causing hypercalcaemia. Any patient being treated with both medications should have their serum calcium measured on a regular basis to prevent excessively high levels of calcium in the body. Thiazides also produce a similar drug interaction when used in conjunction with vitamin D; therefore patients taking calcium and vitamin D with thiazides should be monitored closely to check for signs of hypercalcaemia. This may mean that the therapy requires to be altered or even discontinued with respect to calcium or vitamin D.[13]

References

1. Royal College of Physicians. *Osteoporosis. Clinical Guidelines for Prevention and Treatment.* London: Royal College of Physicians, 1999.
2. Kanis J A. The use of calcium in the management of osteoporosis. *Bone* 1999; 24: 279–290.

3. Elders P J, Netelenbos J C, Lips P, *et al*. Calcium supplementation reduces vertebral bone loss. *J Clin Endocrinol Metab* 1991; **73**: 533–540.

4. Woolf A D, Dixon A S. *Osteoporosis: a Clinical Guide*. London: Martin Dunitz, 1988.

5. Kanis J A. *Osteoporosis*. Oxford: Blackwell Science, 1997.

6. Reid I R, Ames R W, Evans M C, *et al*. Effect of calcium supplementation on bone loss in postmenopausal women. *N Engl J Med* 1993; **328**: 460–464.

7. Prevention and treatment of osteoporosis. *MeReC Bull* 1999; **10**: 25–28.

8. Reid I R, Ames R W, Evans M C, *et al*. Long-term effects of calcium supplementation on bone loss and fractures in postmenopausal women a randomised control trial. *Am J Med* 1995; **98**: 331–335.

9. *British National Formulary* No. 46. London: British Medical Association and Royal Pharmaceutical Society, 2003.

10. South African Medical Association – Osteoporosis Working Group. Osteoporosis clinical guideline. *S Afr Med J* 2000; **90**: 907–944.

11. Chapuy M C, Arlot M E, Duboeuf F, *et al*. Vitamin D and calcium to prevent hip fractures in elderly women. *N Engl J Med* 1992; **327**: 1637–1642.

12. Tilyard M W, Spears G F S, *et al*. Treatment of post-menopausal osteoporosis with calcitriol or calcium. *N Engl J Med* 1992; **326**: 357–362.

13. LaCroix A Z, Ott S M, Ichikawa L, *et al*. Low dose hydrochlorothiazide and preservation of bone mineral density in older adults. *Ann Intern Med* 2000; **133**: 516–526.

9

Hormone replacement therapy

The main role of the sex hormones is to maintain sexual function and to determine the physical sexual characteristics. Until recently, it was thought that any other role these hormones might play was minor and one that did not greatly impinge on the general health of the individual. It is now known that this is far from the truth. The sex hormones burst on to the scene during puberty and bring about the maturity of the sex organs, along with the expected physical changes as the adult form develops. The level of the sex hormones within the body then remains relatively constant for the reproductive years. In men, as maturity passes into ageing, there is a slow, but gradual reduction in the male sex hormone testosterone, whereas in women there is a rapid decrease in both oestrogen and progesterone once menstruation has ceased. This period in a woman's life is known as the menopause; once the menopause is complete, the female sex hormones continue to decline, but at a much slower rate.

Menopause

Although there have been claims that men go through a period in their life that simulates the female menopause, the evidence has yet to be found to substantiate this scenario. In the male, there is no corresponding rapid reduction in the level of the sex hormones, therefore it is safe to say that the menopause is an exclusively female event during which there are a number of changes within the body. The majority of women now commence the process of the menopause as they enter later life, since life expectancy, in general, extends much beyond the span to the menopause. This has not always been so, and in the last 200 years the percentage of women going through the menopause has increased significantly.

Most women enter the menopause somewhere between the ages of 45 and 55, the age being determined by both genetic factors and socio-economic status. The menopause is not an overnight event and can last anything from a year up to 11 years, although the usual time scale is about four years. The menopause usually starts with irregular menstruation, both in quality and quantity, with further deterioration until amenorrhoea is reached.

During the initial phase of the menopause the levels of oestrogen and progesterone in the body reduce dramatically; this is counteracted by an increase in the levels of the gonadotrophins, follicle-stimulating hormone (FSH) and luteinising hormone (LH). The gonadotrophins continue to increase in concentration – FSH more so than LH – for a few years after the menopause so that this ratio of the concentrations of the two hormones is always greater than 1. Following this phase, the levels of the two hormones slowly decrease, maintaining the ratio but never reaching the low levels found prior to the menopause.

Before the menopause the female body's main source of oestrogen is the ovaries, particularly in the potent form of oestradiol. The other main source of oestradiol is the adipose tissue, where it is formed as a result of the metabolism of oestrone and androgens. After the menopause there is only a residual production of oestradiol from the ovaries, and so the main source becomes the adipose tissue, from the conversion of androgens. The amount of adipose tissue a woman has will determine the efficiency of the conversion of androgen to oestradiol; an obese woman will produce up to four times more oestradiol from androgen than a woman of normal weight.[1]

Menopausal changes

During the menopause a number of body functions and structural changes occur as a result of the rapid loss of sex hormone production. These body systems which are affected include the genital–urinary, somatic, vasomotor, psychological, skeletal and cardiovascular systems (see Diagnostic Focus, below).[2]

Genital–urinary

Physical and tissue changes in the structure of a number of organs, mainly within the reproductive system, cause changes in the ability to function normally. The epithelium of the vagina becomes thinner and drier, as seen by the altered cytology. This is in part related to the reduction in vaginal secretions, which elevates the pH, leaving the tissue easily traumatised and thus more susceptible to infection.

Other changes include atrophy of the vagina and loss of muscle tone of the pelvic musculature and smaller vulva. The bladder and

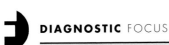

List of body systems affected and disorders arising from the female menopause

Body system	Symptoms/disorders
Autonomic	Hot flushes Sweats Palpitations
Psychological	Mood changes Insomnia Anxiety Depression Impaired memory Impaired concentration
Reproductive tract	Atrophic vaginitis Dyspareunia Reduction of libido
Urinary	Urethral syndrome
Musculoskeletal	Loss of muscle bulk Osteoporosis Thin skin
Cardiovascular	Coronary heart disease

urethra are also affected leading to the likelihood of stress incontinence, prolapse and cystitis.

Somatic

The lower levels of oestrogen in the body during the menopause leads to the skin becoming thinner, with a subsequent loss of strength and elasticity; the collagen content is reduced and the overall effect of all these factors is the natural ageing of the skin seen in women of menopausal age. A severe reduction of oestrogen and a corresponding increase in androgens can produce a male pattern of baldness, together with a hirsute facial appearance.

The incidence of heart disease in women changes as they proceed to the menopause, ranging from a condition rarely seen to one of known consequence in the female population. The prevalence of heart disease in postmenopausal women is similar to that of men; the difference is the change in lipid profile to a higher concentration of cholesterol, triglycerides and low-density lipoproteins. Thus, the risk factors of postmenopausal women developing ischaemic heart disease are increased, bringing their proclivity to such illness in to line with that of men.

Vasomotor

A frequent symptom of the menopause is the commonly called 'hot flush', which may affect up to 75% of women. The redness and flushing can occur throughout the body, but in most cases is confined to the neck and face, usually lasting for about 4 minutes. The flushing of the skin is associated with a distinct elevation in skin temperature, a reduction in body temperature, and with a transient tachycardia. There is a reflex increase in sweating during the period of the flush, which can be particularly disturbing at night.

Psychological

The many changes that the body is undergoing during the period leading up to the menopause can give rise to a number of psychological symptoms: whether the symptoms are a direct effect of these changes or a consequence of becoming postmenopausal is open to debate. The connected depression, insomnia, irritability, premenstrual mood swings and loss of concentration could be said to be a consequence of the menopausal activity, whereas loss of libido and sexual activity could be due to the direct result of changes in the vagina following the reduction in oestrogen.

Skeletal

The symptoms of change within the various body systems during the menopause are largely self-evident and occur within a defined period; the exception to this is the skeleton, where the gradual process of change goes on unnoticed. The effects on the skeleton cause the greatest morbidity, as they can produce a profound difference in the quality of life, with detrimental changes in socio-economic status.

The gradual loss of bone mass from peak bone mass caused by ageing is accelerated at the time of the menopause because of the reduced oestrogen production level. Bone loss returns closer to a rate similar to that prior to the menopause and may even become slower, depending on the level of the remaining bone mass.

There are a number of factors that can influence the rate and extent of bone mass loss, most of which relate to the formation of the bones and the peak bone mass achieved. The female sex hormones play a pivotal role in the production of bone within the skeleton, and anything that reduces or enhances these hormones will have an effect on bone formation and loss. Peak bone mass can be augmented by maintaining a reasonable level of physical activity during the reproductive years. Use of oral contraceptives for more than six months and multiple births will increase bone mass by reducing bone loss. Bone loss may be increased by a late menarche and an early menopause, and by periods of amenorrhoea brought on by excessive physical exercise or starvation dieting; this reduces production of sex hormones, thus mimicking the menopause.

It is well known that the lack of oestrogen will cause loss of bone mass from patients who have experienced an early surgical menopause because of removal of the ovaries. It is standard practice to give such patients hormone replacement therapy (HRT), following the removal of the major source of oestrogen production.

An individual's risk of bone fracture is determined by the amount and type of bone loss. As discussed earlier, there are two types of bone – cortical and trabecular — and the degree of bone loss from each type will predict the risk of fracture. Trabecular bone comprises the structural part of the bone and provides the main strength; therefore, loss from this area quickly causes the individual to become prone to fracture risk. Cortical bone gives support to the main structure of trabecular bone, and thus more cortical bone can be lost before fracture risk is comparable with that resulting from loss of trabecular bone.

Exactly how the lack of oestrogen reduces bone mass is unclear. There is a theory that oestrogen mediates the uptake of calcium into the bone. Evidence of this is the presence of oestrogen receptors within the nucleus of oesteoblast-like cells.[3]

Cardiovascular

The menopause alters lipid metabolism from one producing a beneficial mixture of lipoproteins and cholesterol, into one where there is an increase in total cholesterol and low-density lipoproteins, although the high-density lipoproteins remain roughly the same. These alterations in the lipid profile are coupled to increases in fibrinogen, plus some clotting factors, which bring with them an increased risk of atheroma, leading to a higher risk of cardiovascular disease.[4]

Menopausal changes in calcium balance

In the early stages of the menopause there is a reduction in the amount of vitamin D in the serum, which leads to a reduced ability to absorb calcium. This, in fact, may be a precursor to the malabsorption of calcium in the postmenopausal period, because the presence of vitamin D is necessary for absorption of calcium from the intestine. The greater need for calcium in the body after the menopause can be attributed to a poor absorption rate and the increased loss of calcium from bone.

It is thought that the loss of oestrogen is responsible for this reduction in vitamin D levels and hence alteration in the absorption of calcium. There is an alternative theory that the lack of oestrogen could have a direct effect on bone, causing it to liberate calcium into the extracellular fluid (ECF). Excessive calcium in the ECF will suppress the secretion of the parathyroid hormone and the synthesis of vitamin D, hence the malabsorption of calcium from the intestine.

Independent of the menopause, there appears to be an age-related reduction of vitamin D, which may be associated with an increase in the secretion of the parathyroid hormone. The gradual impairment of renal function that occurs with age could account for this, as these changes exist in both osteoporotic and non-osteoporotic patients. There are, therefore, a number of possible mechanisms underlying the change in the calcium balance, many of which are both directly and indirectly linked to the menopause.[5]

Drug therapy

Oestrogen was first discovered in 1923 as a separate chemical entity, and this led to the synthesis of the related compounds ethinylestradiol and diethylstilbestrol by 1938. Following further developments of synthetic and semisynthetic oestrogens in the 1950s, clinical studies were undertaken to evaluate their use. At this stage, the use of oestrogen on a long-term basis was observed to have benefits in the maintenance of stature in postmenopausal women. However, there was no sensitive test with which to evaluate these effects until the 1960s, when single photon absorptiometry and radiogrammetry were developed, capable of measuring bone mass and allowing investigation into the full effects on the skeleton. The use of oestrogen replacement therapy was then promoted, not only for the benefits on the skeleton, but also for the relief of the postmenopausal symptoms. This treatment continued until the mid-1970s, when it was discovered that the use of oestrogen therapy added an extra risk factor for the development of endometrial carcinoma. At the same time, further evidence from long-term studies confirmed the skeletal benefits and provided a valid reason for continued therapy.

Despite this major benefit of oestrogen therapy, confidence in its use fell dramatically because of the link with endrometrial carcinoma. In an effort to allay fears, research was conducted to discover if the risk could be reduced. This led to the discovery that a combination of oestrogen and progestogen in similar proportions to that found in menstruating women had the desired effect without the additional risk. This is now the basis of the present-day combination sex HRT for post-menopausal women.[6]

HRT in women has until recently been used only as a short-term measure for natural menopause, although it has been used as a long-term therapy in women with surgical menopause. The evidence of long-term benefits obtained from women who had undergone a surgical menopause led to today's use of HRT as a prolonged therapy in women after a natural menopause. This preventative use of HRT in post-menopausal women has been studied further to establish the optimum course length, timing and combination regimens.

The medicinal products available have been modified in both the dosage and the presentation, in an attempt to make them more acceptable to end-users. This has taken the simple loose tablets, which were the initial format, through an evolution into calendar packs of numerous varieties using colour and novel dispensers to aid patient compliance. In tandem, there has been an interest in developing different pharmaceutical forms, such as transdermal patches and implants having variable rates of drug delivery. The modern pharmaceutical forms have been produced in an effort to enable dose reductions, because of the more selective drugs in use and to minimise drug side-effects. Similarly, new drugs have been researched, with the aim of achieving a more specific role, together with a reduction in side-effects and enhanced patient compliance.[5]

Treating the menopause

The physical difficulties that accompany a woman's passage through the menopause are extremely variable, fluctuating from mild transient symptoms with little effect on lifestyle, to long-lasting symptoms severe enough to disrupt the normal activities of daily life. Women who experience symptoms severe enough to alter their quality of life are highly likely to seek medical advice because of their inability to cope with regular work or social roles. In these cases, treatment is commonly sought for the short-term relief of physical changes in the genital–urinary, vasomotor and somatic body systems. It is because women at this stage select themselves for treatment that is based on the severity of the short-term symptoms, rather than the possibility of long-term benefits, that they often discontinue therapy within one or two years when they feel there is no further benefit.

Following surgical menopause where the uterus and ovaries have been removed it is routine for oestrogen replacement therapy to be prescribed as a matter of course. The intention with this therapy is that it should be continued for a prolonged period, nominally in the order of ten years. The oestrogen is seen as a necessary supplement because the natural source has been removed and it is required to maintain normal function.

The use of HRT in these two differing ways for the treatment of symptoms resulting from the two main causes of the female menopause – natural and surgical – has been the norm until recently. The evidence of benefits from the use of HRT in the surgical menopause patients has led to its more widespread use in natural menopausal women. This has encouraged research into the reasons why HRT should have all the advantages seen in later life for postmenopausal women, in particular in symptomless conditions.

Symptomatic control

Some of the most distressing symptoms of the menopause are caused by vasomotor instability; this is the origin of the hot flushes and sweats related to the lower level of oestrogen. These symptoms are controlled by oestrogen replacement therapy. Similarly, the genital–urinary disorders of vaginal dryness, leading to painful intercourse, are relieved with oestrogen supplements, as are repeated urinary tract infections, although incontinence is not affected by replacement therapy. The psychological problems connected with the menopause are in some way relieved by the sense of well-being achieved through the resolution of the physical symptoms, but it may also be that oestrogen therapy has a direct effect, by restoring hormone levels again to the normal physiological range.[5]

Skeletal effects of hormone replacement

The use of oestrogen after the menopause has a direct effect on bone, by reducing the elevated bone turnover brought about by the onset of the menopause. This immediately reduces the body's demand for calcium by conserving calcium within the bone. There is also a slowing down of the rate of bone loss, since activity within the bone is reduced, therefore the demand for other raw materials used in the process of bone remodelling is decreased.

In this way, the use of oestrogen has been shown to maintain bone mass, retain bone strength and maintain posture. To some extent, progesterone also has a role in reducing bone mass. Advances in the ability to measure bone density have consolidated the evidence for the beneficial effects of both oestrogen and progesterone in various parts of the skeleton. Depending on the stage of introduction, HRT may not only be seen to have the effect of arresting any loss of bone mass, but may even lead to an increase in bone mass.[5]

Effects of HRT on fracture risk

Although enhancement of bone mass is advantageous, the main aim of therapy in osteoporosis is the reduction of fracture rate. Hence studies that confirm a lower rate of fractures in the hip and wrist in post-menopausal women who have been given HRT will further confirm the value of the intervention in this context. The changes in posture seen in osteoporosis are lessened by the use of HRT, as there is a decrease in vertebral fractures and loss of vertebral height. The reduction of risk of osteoporotic fractures in postmenopausal women is dependent on the stage at which the replacement therapy is commenced – the earlier the better.[7,8]

Choice of drug and dose

The choice of drug and formulation is primarily influenced by the causes of the menopause; as discussed earlier, women who have had a surgical menopause require oestrogen-only replacement therapy, whereas women who have gone through a non-surgical menopause require combined replacement therapy, because of a reduced rate of production of oestrogen and progesterone.

Preparations used in oestrogen therapy are produced either from natural oestrogens, such as estradiol and estrone, or synthetic oestrogens, such as ethinylestradiol. Synthetic oestrogens have fallen out of favour because of the superior ability of natural oestrogen to more closely mimic the profile required for HRT. The commonly prescribed conjugated equine oestrogen has a similar profile to the natural human oestrogen.

The oral dose of oestrogen necessary to produce a beneficial effect on bone density has been shown to be about 625 μg conjugated oestrogen, 1–2 mg estradiol. This produces the correct concentration in the body to minimise bone loss and in some cases to restore bone mass. In all cases, the dose given should be monitored against the expected response, which ought to be changes in bone density. Although oestrogen levels can be measured, they rarely are!

In women who have undergone a non-surgical menopause and who have an intact uterus, it is now advocated that a progestogen is given in combination, in order to reduce the possible risk of endometrial carcinoma. Progestogens are available as a number of different drugs, namely norethisterone, dydrogesterone, medroxyprogesterone, levonorgestrel and progesterone. There are two different regimens for using progestogens: combined sequential, where a progestogen is given for 12–14 days of the cycle, and combined continuous, where it is given for the complete cycle. The advantage of the combined continuous regimen is that after about 4–6 months, no breakthrough bleeding occurs within the cycle (see Management Focus, below).[9]

Route of administration

The traditional method of administering HRT, whether it is oestrogen only or the combination of oestrogen and a progestogen, is as an oral

MANAGEMENT FOCUS

Different formulations of hormone replacement therapy			
	Oestrogen only	*Combined sequential*	*Combined continuous*
Hormone	Oestrogen	Oestrogen + progestogen for 12–14 days of cycle	Oestrogen + progestogen continuously
Intact uterus present	No	Yes	Yes
Timing	During/after menopause	During/after menopause	After menopause
Bleeding characteristics	Not applicable	Withdrawal bleeding after progestogen	Spotting for first 4–6 months, then no bleeding

medication in the form of tablets. Until recently, these tablets were presented as loose tablets, but today they are now commonly presented in a strip pack, with directions on when to take them in order to aid compliance. The strip pack is often laid out to coincide with a calendar month and the more complex regimens have been simplified, with the tablets laid out in such a manner as to direct the patient when to take each tablet. There is even a device that delivers a tablet each day through an open slot created by breaking a seal. Once the seal has been broken, subsequent tablets are obtained by positioning the opening over the next available tablet.

In the past few years, a number of novel pharmaceutical delivery devices have been introduced for prolonged administration of a drug; the transdermal skin patch is one of these. The transdermal skin patch has been used to deliver HRT for up to seven days per patch, though the usual period of use of each patch is 3–4 days. There are also gels, which are applied to certain areas of the body: arms, shoulders or inner thighs. The gel is allowed to dry on the skin over a period of five minutes, during which it must not to be touched, or come in to contact with the clothes; a further hour should elapse before contact is made with another human being, particularly male.

Oestrogen can be administered in the form of an estradiol implant placed under the skin for a period of 4–8 months. It is good practice to check oestrogen blood levels prior to each implant, as this will determine the time interval for each implant. This means that the patient will need to visit a specialist clinic, not only for the insertion of the implant, but also for the monitoring, which is usually undertaken within a hospital setting. Because such a method of administration is less convenient, even though carried out only twice a year, it is reserved for those patients intolerant to or non-compliant with other forms of medication. [9]

Timing of replacement therapy

Prior to the commencement of HRT, the woman should be thoroughly examined for any early signs or pre-existing symptoms of either breast or endometrial carcinoma. At the same time, the woman should be counselled with regard to the full benefits of the therapy, as well as the risks, plus an explanation of the monitoring needed to minimise these risks (see Risk Factor Focus, below).

Information should be given on all the various preparations available, in order to enable the woman to choose the one that most suits her particular lifestyle.

RISK FACTOR FOCUS

Contraindications to hormone replacement therapy	
Severity of risk	Contraindications
Absolute	Breast carcinoma
	Endometrial carcinoma (oestrogen-dependent)
	Endometrial hyperplasia
Relative	Myocardial infarction
	Cerebrovascular accident
	Thromboembolic disease
	Familial hyperlipidaemia
	Liver disease
	Breast dysplasia or family history of breast carcinoma
	Hypertension
	Obesity
	Heavy smoking
	Oestrogen-dependent pelvic disease
	Fibroids
	Endometriosis
	Malignant melanoma
	Acute intermittent porphyria
	Severe migraine

Once the risks factors of HRT have been assessed and explained, the aims of the therapy should be discussed and how it will affect and control the menopausal symptoms, in both the short and long term. The side-effects of the treatment must be made clear, especially those that may lead a patient to become either non-compliant or to discontinue the therapy, for example: nausea, vomiting, abdominal discomfort, bloating, weight gain, breast enlargement or tenderness, premenstrual syndrome, fluid retention, depression, headache or migraine. If any of these side-effects do occur, a further discussion with the woman will be required in order to reassess the situation and determine the way forward, either by continuing the current medication or changing the formulation to a different preparation.

Usually, the compelling reason a woman seeks medical advice at the onset of the menopause is to obtain relief from the acute vasomotor symptoms, in particular, hot flushes and sweats. It is at this stage that the woman requires counselling to enable her to decide on her future course of action and whether HRT is suitable for her at this time. Much will depend on the age of the woman on entering the menopause; other aspects to be considered will include any family history of osteoporosis, breast or endometrial carcinoma.

Once it has been decided to prescribe HRT, the next step is to decide what form of preparation is needed. If the woman has an intact uterus, then combination therapy will be prescribed, rather than oestrogen alone. If she is either still going through the menopause or within a few years of ceasing menstrual activity, then the combined sequential therapy should be given. Continuous combined HRT is only indicated at least three years after the menopause.

HRT is very effective against vasomotor symptoms, relieving hot flushes in 95% of women. Hot flushes and sweats will be eased within two weeks of starting therapy; other related symptoms may take a little longer. The maximum therapeutic effect of any dosage form is normally attained within a three-month period. Insufficient control of symptoms after this time suggests that the dose should be increased, if possible, or an alternative formulation chosen. Having achieved the optimum relief of postmenopausal symptoms with the replacement therapy, this treatment should be continued for a few years to prevent re-occurrence of the symptoms. The major reason why HRT is discontinued at this stage is because there is no further perception of benefit.

The use of HRT in this way for just a few years will confer only a short-term benefit – the relief of the acute vasomotor symptoms. On discontinuation of the therapy any long-term benefits, such as prevention of bone loss and cardiac protection, are quickly reversed. It is known that in order to maintain the reduced risk of fracture the minimum period of use is five years, but more likely to be 7–10 years. Women who are prepared to continue to take a form of combined HRT for more than just a few years have the option of switching to continuous combined HRT. The major advantage of this is that after a few months breakthrough bleeding ceases as the continuous progestogen blocks menstruation. This can be an aid to patient compliance, as the lack of a menstrual bleed is often seen as an advantage of being postmenopausal.

Continued use of HRT over a number of years must be monitored carefully and dosage of the two hormones should be altered accordingly, normally by reducing the dose to minimise side-effects. There is a school of thought that advocates having a break from HRT for just a few months or, in the case of prolonged use, a few years, or alternatively restricting use to the period of life when a woman is most likely to experience the possible detrimental effects of osteoporosis, that is after the age of sixty.[8]

Cessation of hormone therapy

The usual reason for HRT being discontinued is that the woman is no longer willing to tolerate the side-effects. This sometimes happens when the aims of the therapy have not been discussed fully and put into the context of the short- and long-term benefits of the treatment. Non-compliance can occur within the first few months of the woman commencing the HRT, just at the point when the short-term benefits are about to be realised; however symptoms will re-occur shortly after the medication has been stopped. In such circumstances, the woman has often made up her mind that the side-effects are worse than the symptoms of the menopause.

If the HRT is started shortly after or during the menopause for the relief of the vasomotor symptoms, then the course length should be in the order of 2–3 years. At the initial assessment, a decision should be made with regard to the level of benefit to be experienced by the patient from the longer term use of the supplements. This should depend on whether the woman is at risk of osteoporosis or cardio-vascular disease, either from a previous family history or predisposing risk factors.

The use of HRT should be monitored closely, particularly in cases where the menopause has occurred early and a prolonged use of the therapy – of up to or exceeding ten years – is envisaged. If the menopause is experienced before the age of 45, then the ten-year period would be completed well before the age of 60, when the replacement therapy would yield the greatest benefit. In the case of an early menopause, where a long period of HRT is required, monitoring every 6–12 months for early signs of breast or endometrium carcinoma is essential. The HRT should be continued as long as the bone mineral density measurements remain consistent. When the bone mineral density starts to fall, despite the HRT, a reassessment must be made to determine whether to continue the current therapy or the current therapy plus an additional therapy, or to switch to an alternative therapy.

HRT can be started at any stage after the menopause, especially if there is a need for protection against bone fracture. In a woman beginning therapy later in life, in the seventh decade or beyond, it may be more beneficial to start on a lower dose to avoid troublesome side-effects, such as breast tenderness. These women may need closer monitoring in the initial stages of therapy to confirm that the benefit-to-risk ratio is in the woman's favour.[8]

HRT combined with other drugs

In order to achieve the maximum benefit from HRT it is necessary to ensure that the woman obtains adequate nutrition, particularly with respect to calcium and vitamin D. Frequently, the level of both calcium and vitamin D is not optimised, therefore supplementation, especially of calcium of between 10 and 20 mmol, dependent on diet, gives additional benefits.

Recently, other drugs, such as bisphosphonates, have been combined with HRT in the treatment of osteoporosis. In the few studies that have been carried out in this field it has been shown that the bisphosphonates do provide added benefit to HRT, owing to the different mode of action.

Non-skeletal aspects of oestrogen therapy

HRT been shown to have a beneficial effect not only in osteoporosis, but also in a number of other medical conditions such as cardiovascular disease, stroke, venous thromboembolism, glucose and lipid metabolism.

Cardiovascular disease

It has been known for a number of years that a woman who is still menstruating has a low risk of cardiovascular disease, the inference being that oestrogen protects women up to the start of the menopause. After the menopause, the level of cardiovascular disease in women becomes equal to that in men; in later life the incidence in women actually exceeds that in men.

Therefore, if postmenopausal women are given HRT then this should convey a cardioprotective effect and reduce cardiac events to the same level as that in premenopausal women. This simple hypothesis has not worked out in practice and in fact there seems to be a more complex relationship between HRT and cardiovascular disease.

The results from a long-term study involving more than 70 000 women showed that women who have taken HRT have a 40% reduction in non-fatal heart attacks and fatal heart conditions compared with women who have never taken HRT.[10] This result did not depend either on dosage or whether the preparation was oestrogen-only or oestrogen with progestogen. The cardiovascular advantage of HRT was maintained for up to ten years before the benefit rapidly diminished.

Another clinical study of women with pre-existing cardiovascular disease showed that there was no benefit from the introduction of HRT.

Neither the content of the therapy, nor the amount of the relative dosages appeared to influence the result. However, the validity of this clinical trial has been questioned, both with regard to the preparations used and the age group of the subjects.[11,12]

Cerebrovascular events

There has been conflicting evidence concerning the possible increase in the risk of cerebrovascular events, such as stroke, during or after the use of HRT. A clinical study that examined high doses of oestrogen demonstrated an increased risk, whereas a meta-analysis failed to prove a link.[12]

Venous thromboembolism

There is an increased risk of venous thromboembolism associated with HRT. This is related to the oestrogen content and is independent of progestogen dosage. Although the overall risk is still low – the risk rises from 10 per 100 000 in non-users to 30 per 100 000 in users and the mortality rate for sufferers is about 1–2% – the recommendation from the Committee on Safety of Medicines is that caution should be used in the prescribing of HRT in women with predisposing factors for venous thromboembolism.[12]

Glucose and lipid metabolism

Oestrogen has been shown to increase high-density lipoprotein (HDL) cholesterol and to reduce low-density lipoprotein (LDL) cholesterol, promoting a cardioprotective lipid profile. Progestogens can antagonise this beneficial effect of oestrogen, particularly levonorgestrel, norethisterone and medroxyprogesterone; but progesterone and dydrogesterone have a neutral effect.

In addition, oestrogen has a beneficial effect on the decrease in insulin resistance that can be present in later life. Again, the progestogens counteract this advantageous effect on glucose metabolism to a varying degree.

Breast cancer

The Committee on Safety of Medicines reviewed the incidence of breast cancer as an adverse effect of long-term HRT. The data would indicate that the longer a woman is taking HRT, the greater the risk of breast cancer. Obviously, if a woman uses HRT for relief of the menopausal symptoms and discontinues therapy within months of commencing then there is very little increased risk of breast cancer. If the woman has taken HRT for a number of years, then the risk is much greater; but on stopping the therapy, this risk diminished to the extent that five years from cessation the increased risk is negligible when compared with that of non-users of HRT.

A brief review of the figures gives a better impression of the degree of risk that is run with the use of HRT. After five years, the risk of breast cancer is comparable with that of non-users. Even at ten years, the risk has only increased to around 0.5% greater than that of those women not taking HRT. At 15 years, the risk has doubled to reach over just 1% greater than those women who have not taken HRT.

The increase risk of breast cancer with HRT is related to tumours that have oestrogen receptors and are activated by the excess oestrogen in the HRT. Therefore, if a therapy were produced that did not activate the oestrogen receptors in the breast tissue, then the level of risk in both groups of women would be the same.[12,13]

Selective oestrogen receptor modulators (SERM)

The first drug from this group, raloxifene, was introduced because it was believed that, being selective, it would prove to have less of a risk of breast cancer than HRT. This was proved to be the case when a large clinical trial of raloxifene, known as Multiple Outcomes of Raloxifene Evaluation (MORE), was carried out. This found that the raloxifene did not activate the oestrogen receptors involved in breast cancer, but the major disadvantage was an increase in the incidence of venous thrombo-embolism.

Other drugs within this group are in the process of being evalu-ated, however results are awaited to ascertain whether they have similar side-effects, particularly concerning venous thromboembolism.[14]

References

1. Studd J W W, Chakravarti S, Oram D. Practical problems in the treatment of the climacteric syndrome. *Postgrad Med J* 1976; **52** (Suppl 6): 60–64.
2. Rees M, Purdie D W. *Management of the menopause: the handbook of the British Menopause Society.* London: BMS Publications, 2002.
3. Hansen M, Overgaard K, Riis B, Christiansen C. Role of peak bone mass and bone loss in postmenopausal osteoporosis: 12 year study. *BMJ* 1991; **303**: 961–964.

4. Woolf A D, Dixon A S. *Osteoporosis: a Clinical Guide*. London: Martin Dunitz, 1988.

5. Kanis J A. *Osteoporosis*. Oxford: Blackwell Science, 1997.

6. Riman T, Dickman P, Nilsson S, *et al*. Hormone replacement therapy and the risk of invasive epithelial ovarian cancer in Swedish women. *J Natl Cancer Inst* 2002; **94**: 497–504.

7. Villareal D T, Binder E F, Williams D B, *et al*. Bone mineral density response to estrogen replacement in frail elderly women. *JAMA* 2001; **286**: 815–820.

8. Torgerson D J, Bell-Syer S E M. Hormone replacement therapy and prevention of nonvertebral fractures. *JAMA* 2001; **285**: 2891–2897.

9. *British National Formulary* No. 46. London: British Medical Association and Royal Pharmaceutical Society, 2003.

10. Grodstein F, Manson J E, Colditz G A. A prospective, observational study of postmenopausal hormone therapy and primary prevention of cardiovascular disease. *Ann Intern Med* 2000; **133**: 933–941.

11. Hulley S, Grady D, Bush T, *et al*. Randomised trial of estrogen and progestin for secondary prevention of coronary heart disease in postmenopausal women. *JAMA* 1998; **280**: 605–613.

12. Committee on Safety of Medicines. Safety update on long-term HRT. *Current Problems in Pharmacovigilance* 2002; **28**: 11–12.

13. Chen C, Weiss N S, Newcomb P, *et al*. Hormone replacement therapy in relation to breast cancer. *JAMA* 2002; **287**: 734–741.

14. Barrett-Connor E, Grady B, Sashegyi A, *et al*. Raloxifene and cardiovascular events in osteoporotic postmenopausal women. *JAMA* 2002; **287**: 847–857.

10

Bisphosphonates

The search for a treatment that improves or reverses bone loss during the natural ageing process has led to research into a number of drugs in varying dosages. One of the more successful of these has been the bisphosphonates, which were first used 20 years ago as a research tool in a last ditch attempt to reduce hypercalcaemia of malignancy. Following success in this area, the research continued in an effort to find further therapeutic roles for these drugs, for example in the treatment of Paget's disease.

At this stage only an injectable form of the drug was available, which was not conducive to long-term therapy. It was not until disodium etidronate was formulated as an oral medication in the form of a tablet given once a day, that routine administration could be tried in order to establish the benefits. From this, came the first application of these drugs as an aid to helping to prevent the bones becoming brittle and fracturing in the treatment of Paget's disease. This therapeutic advance in one bone condition where brittle bones and fractures are a problem inspired researchers to anticipate similar results in the treatment of osteoporosis.[1]

Theoretical basis of bone loss

As stated in previous chapters, bone is not a rigid structure, but a dynamic system in which bone is continually being remodelled. In the body there are two cell types that control bone mass: osteoclasts, which control bone resorption through mineralisation, and osteoblasts, which produce new bone. These processes work in opposition and which one is in the ascendancy determines whether the bone is in a net gain or net loss situation. During the growth years, the activity of the osteoblasts exceeds that of the osteoclasts until peak bone mass is achieved, which usually occurs during the third decade. For a short period the two processes neutralise each other, resulting in a fairly constant bone density; then, under the control of the osteoblasts, there is a gradual and progressive increase in bone resorption and mineralisation. At this period

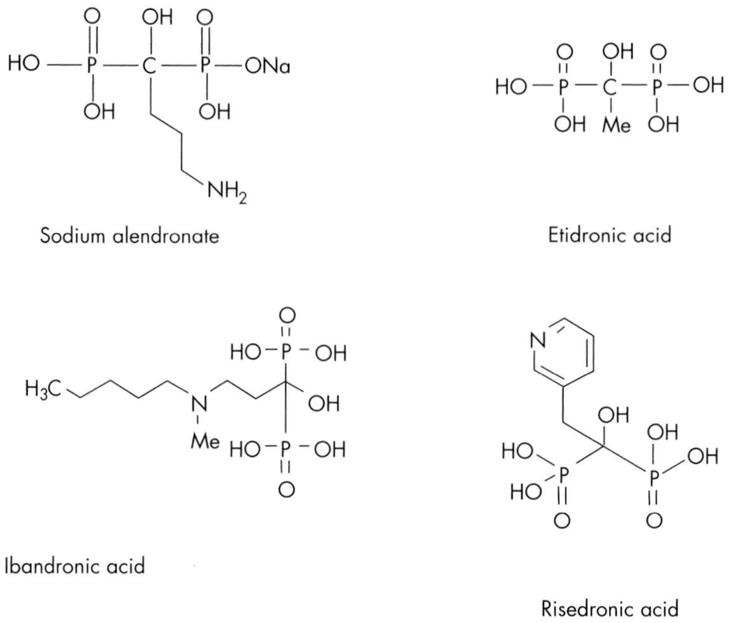

Figure 10.1   The bisphosphonates.

of life, the osteoclasts are unable to keep pace with the osteoblasts, and there is a reduction in the amount of new bone formed, leading to a net bone loss. In order to correct this imbalance, an attempt may be made to increase new bone production or alternatively to try to block the process of bone resorption and bone mineralisation.

In striving to understand the process of bone loss, researchers endeavoured to reverse this action by attempting to promote an increase in bone mass. Unfortunately, although there have been some short-term gains, these were not sustained in the long term. Therefore, instead of promoting new bone production methods, researchers have transferred their attention to the reduction of bone resorption and mineralisation.

The physiological basis for the effect of bisphosphonates on bone is based on the fact that the chemical structure (see Figure 10.1) is similar to that of pyrophosphate. The difference is that instead of the two phosphonates being linked through oxygen, as in the pyrophosphate molecule, the link in bisphosphonates is via a carbon atom with variations on the side-chain. This difference accounts for the ability of the bisphosphonate to bind to bone and is the reason why it is resistant to the normal breakdown by enzymatic hydrolysis present within bone. The creation of a more or less permanent bond between the bisphosphonate and the bone causes an inhibition of skeletal and extraskeletal calcifica-tion, with the inhibition of osteoclast-governed bone resorption, includ-ing inhibition of aortic, renal and dermal calcification induced by vitamin D. Further benefits include the prevention of the calcification of joints arising from changes brought about by arthritis. Bisphosphonates also have the ability, when given in high doses, to inhibit bone mineralisation through the prevention of crystal growth within bone.

There are various drugs within the bisphosphonate group and the differences between them can be predicted, to some extent, by the strength of the bond to the hydroxyapatite crystals in bone. Alteration of the side-chains of the molecular structure of the bisphosphonate can lead to improved binding to bone and enhance the reduction in bone resorption. This modification of the molecular structure of bisphosphon-ates produces drugs that are designed to have a more beneficial effect on bone, by reducing the undesirable effects on mineralisation while at the same time increasing the required effect on bone resorption.

Bisphosphonates achieve their effect on bone resorption by their ability to enter into the osteoclasts, thus altering their permeability to calcium; although this much is known, extensive experimental research has failed to elucidate the actual mechanism by which this occurs. What has been discovered is that bisphosphonates do bind directly to bone at resorption sites, thus blocking the ability of osteoclasts to bind to these sites. This competition at the resorption binding sites between the bisphosphonates and the osteoclasts reduces the potential for resorption, as the bisphosphonates have dominance.

In seeking to identify the specific method by which the bisphosphon-ates produce the known therapeutic effect, animal studies have been designed to elicit individual drug actions on bone at different sites and strengths. These experiments have highlighted differences among some of the drugs within the group. For instance, alendronate binds to resorption sites, whereas etidronate binds to bone formation sites. The variation in the action of these two drugs could be related to the relative amounts taken: the lower doses of alendronate causing binding to the more recep-tive resorption sites, whereas the higher doses of etidronate permit the drug to possibly saturate the resorption sites, leaving the excess drug avail-able to bind to the mineralisation sites of bone formation.

The clinical effect of these mechanisms of drug action is to reduce the action of osteoclasts. This is made evident by the reduction in the depth of the erosion cavities created in the normal process of bone re-modelling. Over a period of time the number of available osteoclasts and the ability to produce them is diminished by the use of bisphosphonates, thus limiting the size and number of the erosion sites; therefore the overall bone remodelling activity is reduced owing to the reduced number of activated bone remodelling sites.[2]

Drug handling

Bisphosphonates are available in both oral and injection forms, but as yet only the oral products have been indicated for the treatment of osteoporosis. A number of difficulties have had to be overcome in the formulation of an oral product, which traditionally has been the pharmaceutical presentation when long-term administration for a chronic condition is required. Initially, drugs discovered and presented as an injection have posed serious problems when being formulated into an oral form, some requiring re-formulation, others never making the transition into an oral form at all.

The main difficulty in producing an oral form of the bisphos-phonates is that the solubility of the drug is low and it possesses a high affinity with calcium, forming insoluble chelates. This low solubility leads to a reduced potential for absorption – anywhere from 0.5% to 10% – depending on the drug, which, coupled with the interaction with calcium, means that it is imperative these drugs are taken on an empty stomach with plenty of fluid, preferably water. The drugs also have an effect on gastric motility, mainly of the upper part of the gastrointestinal tract, but also to a lesser extent on the lower end of the tract, seen as constipation. To reduce these possible effects on absorption, it is rec-ommended that the bisphosphonates be taken first thing in the morning – up to two hours before breakfast, with plenty of water. To prevent upper gastrointestinal problems, particularly in the oesophagus, it is recommended that the patient is standing upright or at least sitting when the drug is administered. The patient should refrain from lying down for 30 minutes afterwards.

Once the drug is absorbed there is a relatively rapid uptake of about 50% into the skeleton, where it binds to bone. This accounts for the short half-life of less than two hours in the circulatory system. There is also some protein binding of the drugs but no detectable binding to soft tissue.

None of the available bisphosphonates have been shown to undergo any degree of metabolism and therefore are eliminated almost exclusively via the kidney unchanged. The half-life of this elimination process is between 6 and 8 hours from the plasma, whereas the elimination half-life from the bone is thought to be anything from a number of weeks to a number of months. Of the absorbed portion, the amount of unchanged drug detected in urine over a 24-hour period can vary from 40% to 80%; the remainder is thought to be bound to bone and eliminated gradually through the process of bone turnover.

The more clinically significant distribution of bisphosphonates is that within the bone, since this is the basis of the pharmacological action of the drugs. There would appear to be an uneven distribution of the drug throughout the affected bone, the drug being attracted to areas of bone where there is the greatest bone loss. This selectivity of the drug to sites where it is most needed is a positive pharmacological advantage, but does present difficulty in estimating the precise dose required to obtain the optimum therapeutic effect. It can lead to focal abnormalities in bone. The clinical significance of this is not known.

The inclusion of bisphosphonates into bone structure by binding to resorption sites in an irreversible way induces a very long half-life of the drug within the skeleton. The duration of the effect of bisphosphonate is further prolonged by the reduction of bone turnover, which in prolonged use can extend a half-life in the bone to weeks or even months. This is particularly evident in osteoporosis, where just a few days of treatment can lead to the drug being still detected in the bone up to a year later. Where bisphosphonates are used in other conditions, although bone retention is high, the therapeutic effect is not sustained for a long period. This could be due to the reduced effect on bone mineralisation in comparison with bone resorption.[2]

Monitoring treatment

In order to prove the effectiveness of the bisphosphonates in the treatment of osteoporosis, further clinical tests and biochemical changes can be undertaken. In general, success is measured by an increase in the bone mass over a 6–12 month period; this provides evidence of restoration of the bone mass, but gives no indication of the strength nor of the state of the underpinning structure. To some extent this will be observed by the monitoring of certain biochemical markers of bone metabolism and resorption, for instance a decrease in urinary hydroxyproline with a knock-on effect seen in serum levels of alkaline phosphatase.

As described previously, the use of bisphosphonates will have the effect of increasing bone formation by inhibiting the process of bone resorption, thus reducing the transport of calcium from bone into extracellular fluid, plasma and eventually urine. Reduction in circulating calcium will lead to a higher level of parathyroid hormone being secreted by the body in an attempt to increase calcium in the blood. A number of drugs exist within the group that bring about these physiological and biochemical changes when used in the treatment of osteoporosis.

The drug etidronate is exceptional in that, when used in low doses of 10–15 mg/kg per day, it increases calcium uptake into the bone from extracellular fluid, conversely when used therapeutically at higher doses of 20 mg/kg per day, while inhibiting bone resorption the beneficial effect on serum and urinary calcium is no longer present. This effect of etidronate has been explained by a dual action of inhibiting bone resorption and the addition of calcium to bone. The adverse effect of etidronate has not been seen with the newer drugs in the group, even after continuous or higher intravenous doses.

The overall result of the therapeutic use of bisphosphonates is that the rate of bone turnover is reduced and shallower erosion cavities are produced. The bone created under these conditions has thicker existing trabecular bone but there is no addition to the amount of trabecular bone.

A number of the bisphosphonates have been shown to be effective in increasing bone mass, however in order to establish the optimum treatment a number of clinical studies have been designed to identify the correct dosage and frequency of drug administration. These studies have shown skeletal bone mass increases in the early part of treatment, which are sustained throughout the first year. In the second year the rate of increase in bone mass is reduced, and this continues as a progression dependent on the severity of the condition at the start of treatment and the drug chosen. What happens after this initial period is again influenced by the choice of drug used in the treatment. Sometimes the initial increase in bone mass ceases and bone loss recommences, but at a slower rate, sometimes the bone mass increase is sustained throughout the treatment, and sometimes bone mass continues to increase during the time of treatment, but at a slower rate in each successive year.[2]

Fracture rate

Although the effectiveness of the bisphosphonates is measured by increased bone mass, proof of this is looked for in the form of a reduction in the incidence of fracture rate – a desired outcome. As previously stated, the bisphosphonates increase bone mass but do not alter bone structure or bone strength. The action of the bisphosphonates appears to maintain rather than increase bone strength and thus the effectiveness of the treatment is dependent on when therapy is commenced.

A number of clinical studies have been undertaken to investigate the decrease in the fracture rate. Initially this was carried out over a relatively short period of 1–2 years, but latterly it was extended to cover longer periods of around five years. Clinical studies have looked at the incidence of vertebral fractures, hip fractures and colles fractures. The incidence of vertebral fractures has been studied extensively using treatment with a number of drugs; in some of these trials loss of height was also measured to further define success of treatment.[3–5]

Bisphosphonates are known to reduce bone pain by reducing bone irregularities, particularly in malignant hypercalcaemia associated with neoplastic disease. This has not yet been extensively studied in osteoporotic fractures, but obvious reduction in fracture rates will be complimented by a reduction in bone pain.[6,7]

Treatment regimens

Bisphosphonates were first introduced as a treatment for osteoporosis using etidronate as a cyclical regimen of 14 days etidronate, 76 days calcium in a three-month period. This was repeated, initially for up to a two-year period, which has now been extended following further clinical trial work. The cyclical regimen initially encountered difficulties in patient compliance, but this has been helped by the production of a combined patient pack of the two medications. Even with these modifications in the presentation and associated information, patients still have problems in complying with (a) the timing of the two treatments and (b) in particular with the palatability of the calcium preparation.

Subsequent oral bisphosphonates have been marketed as a continuous daily treatment regimen and recently alendronate as a continuous weekly regimen, which is seen as an improvement to aid compliance. Currently there are clinical investigations into injectable presentations, which could be given on a monthly, or longer, basis to give sustained therapy with minimal patient effort (see Management Focus, below).[8]

 MANAGEMENT FOCUS

Treatment regimens			
Drug	Regimen	Daily dose	Weekly dose
Etidronate	14 days every 90 days	Yes (for 14 days only)	No
Alendronate	Continuous	Yes	Yes
Risedronate	Continuous	Yes	Yes

Indications for treatment

In women, the commonest reason for the development of osteoporosis is the loss of oestrogen following the menopause. This cohort was therefore the first group to be studied in relation to the use of bisphosphonates as anti-osteoporotic treatment. The first bisphosphonate aimed at the treatment of osteoporosis has been marketed for use in postmenopausal women. In this respect the bisphosphonates are seen as an alternative to hormone replacement therapy (HRT) in women who are unable to tolerate replacement therapy or when hormone treatment is thought to be having no further effect.

Because the incidence of osteoporosis in men is much lower than it is in women, it is much more difficult to obtain sufficient data to show that a particular treatment is effective in halting or reversing the condition in men. This means that it may take a number of years before a new bisphosphonate drug gains an indication for treatment of osteoporosis in men. Bisphosphonates are the foremost form of therapy used in the treatment of osteoporosis in men, because men do not portray the same loss of sex hormones with age and the onset of osteoporosis.[9]

An increasing group of patients requiring treatment for osteoporosis are those who have been prescribed high-dose corticosteroids over a lengthy period of time. The dose in question will have been greater than 7.5 mg prednisolone or its equivalent, taken over a period in excess of three or six months, or alternatively a series of short courses extending over a similar length of time. This treatment leads to a slow progressive loss of bone. Common indications for the use of corticosteroids are asthma, rheumatoid arthritis, inflammatory bowel diseases and a number of skin disorders. All of these conditions, which are chronic, last for many years, during which the patient will be given either short courses of high-dose corticosteroids or lengthy courses of moderate maintenance doses. Each regimen will eventually produce osteoporosis, though it should be noted that a high dose of corticosteroid will rapidly produce bone loss within the first few weeks of treatment.

The bisphosphonates act by reversing some of the adverse effects that corticosteroids have on bone; in particular they inhibit the increase in osteoclast-mediated bone resorption and this helps to compensate for the inhibition of osteoblast activity in bone formation. In this way the bisphosphonates have been shown to prevent corticosteroid bone loss and even bring about a net increase in bone mass.[10]

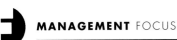

Dosages for prevention and treatment of osteoporosis		
Drug	*Prevention dosage*	*Treatment dosage*
Etidronate	400 mg	400 mg
Alendronate	5 mg daily 10 mg daily (women not on HRT)	10 mg daily 70 mg weekly
Risedronate	5 mg daily 35 mg weekly	5 mg daily 35 mg weekly

Individual drugs

In order to gain a more detailed knowledge of the use of the bisphosphonates in the treatment of osteoporosis it is necessary to look at the drugs within the group on an individual basis. This will explain in detail how the drugs are used clinically and what evidence exists to prove their efficacy. The currently available drugs indicated for treatment of osteoporosis are discussed below in alphabetical order, rather than any other specific precedence. The dosages for prevention and treatment of osteoporosis are summarised in the Management Focus above.

Alendronate

Used in both the treatment and prevention of osteoporosis, alendronate is licensed in the UK for use in postmenopausal women, men and corticosteroid-induced osteoporosis. It is administered as a continuous regimen and the patient is given specific advice to ensure that calcium and vitamin D intakes are high enough to enable the therapy to reach optimum effect. The prevention dosage is 5 mg daily and the treatment dosage in postmenopausal women is 10 mg daily. A recent advance has seen the introduction of the 70 mg dosage administered once per week. The prevention and treatment dosage of 10 mg prescribed for treatment of corticosteroid-induced osteoporosis is given only to women who are not receiving HRT.

The best time of the day for the patient to take the medication is first thing in the morning after rising; the medication should not be taken before bedtime nor in the morning before getting up. The medicine must be taken with a full glass of water on an empty stomach and ideally the patient should be standing up or sitting upright and must remain in an upright position for a further 30 minutes. An interval of at least half an hour must elapse before any food is taken.

The reasons for the patient to take the drug on an empty stomach and to drink a large volume of water are to ensure that there is no inter-action between the drug and any food consumed, while the large volume of fluid taken in an upright position, whether standing or sitting, helps to limit the upper gastrointestinal side-effects on the oesophagus and ensures that the drug dissolution is adequate. The patient being in an upright position enables the tablet to slide down the oesophagus under the influence of gravity, while the large volume of fluid acts as a lubri-cant surrounding the tablet. Unfortunately, even when this advice is followed to the letter some discomfort can arise, originating in the oesophagus where the tablet can adhere to the epithelial lining.[8]

Clinical effectiveness

The use of alendronate in postmenopausal women has shown to be effec-tive in increasing bone mass at a number of sites within the skeleton, namely hip, spine and forearm. This has been seen both in animal studies and in short-term – up to two years – clinical studies. These initial studies led to further investigation into the longer term effects and to establish if alendronate could prevent fracture, a more significant outcome and one necessary to maintain a better quality of life.

To begin with, clinical studies investigated the use of alendronate in postmenopausal women over a period of three years, checking the inci-dence of all types of fracture incurred during the time the patients were receiving treatment. Over the time period there was not only evidence of increase in bone mass but also a 48% reduction in vertebral fractures in comparison with the placebo group. Similarly, there was improvement in the level of progression of vertebral deformities and loss of height.

A dose of 5 mg alendronate has proved to be an effective alterna-tive to HRT for patients who cannot tolerate the side-effects of hormone therapy. In a study that compared the effectiveness of alendronate and HRT, both treatments produced similar improvements in bone mineral density at the spine and hip. In conclusion, alendronate was seen as another option in the prevention of bone loss in postmenopausal women, particularly in women unable to tolerate HRT.

It is important in treating this chronic condition that the available therapy is able to consistently produce results over a long period. The short-term studies of up to three years described above, although promising, needed to be followed up by research lasting in excess of five years. A succession of long-term studies has shown that there are continual benefits to be obtained from the ongoing use of alendronate. These benefits include year on year increases in bone mineral density at the spine and the maintenance of bone mineral density at the hip. This leads to a reduction in the incidence of fractures in women who are taking alendronate for up to seven years.

Further clinical work to demonstrate the effectiveness of alendronate in a variety of osteoporotic conditions has shown that the benefits seen in postmenopausal women are also observed in men and in corticosteroid-induced osteoporosis. This has recently brought about a change in the licensed indications for alendronate, which includes these additional osteoporotic conditions.[7]

Side-effects

The major side-effect of alendronate is upper gastrointestinal irritation, experienced as difficulty in swallowing, new or worsening heartburn, pain on swallowing or retrosternal pain. These symptoms can develop into severe oesophageal reactions such as oesophagitis, oesophageal ulcers, oesophageal stricture and oesophageal erosions. The development of these symptoms would be a reason for discontinuation of the treatment because of the seriousness of the possible reaction. In order to reduce the incidence of these side-effects it is important to follow closely the advised method of administration, that is with plenty of fluid, and for the patient to remain in the upright position for at least 30 minutes after taking the drug.

Other gastrointestinal side-effects include abdominal pain, flatulence, distension, diarrhoea or constipation, nausea, vomiting and peptic ulceration. A transient reduction in serum calcium and phosphate will occur, which is only to be expected knowing the mode of action. Allergic reactions can happen, causing erythema, rash, photosensitivity and even hypersensitivity reactions.[11]

Etidronate

Etidronate was the first bisphosphonate to be introduced initially for the treatment of postmenopausal women, then latterly for use in men and in the treatment of corticosteroid-induced osteoporosis. It is given in a cyclical intermittent regimen in conjunction with calcium. As described earlier, this has been devised following clinical studies to evaluate mode of action and to establish the need for an activation and deactivation period of bone resorption sites. In this way the etidronate prevents bone loss and the calcium increases bone mass as it is taken up into the bone following administration of large doses in excess of normal daily requirements.

The treatment regimen for etidronate comprises 14 days of active therapy and 76 days of calcium. This is available in a combined pack marketed as *Didronel PMO*. The etidronate must be taken on an empty stomach, at least two hours after eating any food, and abstinence from food should be observed for two hours afterwards. The reason for this is that etidronate would bind to any calcium-containing food, for example milk. Antacid mixtures must be avoided, together with iron therapy and mineral supplements because of the chelation of the ions with etidronate. In order to overcome these problems of interaction, particularly with food, it is advised that the etidronate is taken first thing in the morning two hours before breakfast.

The etidronate is taken for 14 days only in the three-month cycle. This is followed by calcium therapy in the form of a soluble tablet that produces an orange fizzy drink. This can be difficult to tolerate; it is described by many patients as being unpalatable.[8]

Clinical effectiveness

The initial clinical studies of etidronate in the early 1990s were the first to show any efficacy in the treatment of osteoporosis in postmenopausal women. At the time, these studies were ground breaking, as they were the first to use bisphosphonates in an oral form in order to demonstrate an increase in bone mass and a decrease in fracture rate. This provoked interest not only in the use of etidronate in osteoporosis, but also in the condition itself, highlighting the extent of the problem and the need for alternative therapies. In the beginning, these short-term studies limited the use of etidronate in patients to two years, until longer term studies had been completed and the use of the drug could be extended.

As etidronate was the first bisphosphonate to be administered on a routine basis because of its availability as an oral preparation, its use in all types of osteoporosis was studied. This development of the drug coincided with an increase in awareness of the incidence and causes of osteoporosis, and etidronate was included in the armoury of treatments for the condition. Further clinical evaluation of the drug's effectiveness resulted in its license for use in the treatment of men with osteoporosis.

The wider use of corticosteroids in the treatment of a number of chronic conditions for periods in excess of 12 months meant that the prevalence of osteoporosis in these patients was increasing. In the majority of cases this was caused by the use of prednisolone, which was the main oral corticosteroid drug prescribed in doses greater than 7.5 mg per day for between three and six months. This treatment regimen can reduce bone mass by up to 5%, which considerably increases the risk of fracture, particularly in older postmenopausal women. The rise in the incidence of osteoporosis in these patients high-lighted the need for a viable therapy to prevent bone mass loss. Cyclical etidronate was thus tried in patients who had received high-dose prednisolone for the last three months and were expected to continue on this treatment for at least a further 12 months. This first clinical trial showed that etidronate over a short period would prevent bone loss in the spine and the hip. The repetition of this clinical trial work with patients who had been taking prednisolone for a number of years prior to treatment produced similar results. Clinical studies lasting for two years then showed that the improvement was progressive, with an expected slower increase in bone mass in the second year. In the longer studies a reduction in fracture rate was identified in patients receiving the active treatment of cyclical etidronate.

This clinical research has established etidronate and other bisphosphonates as a means of preventing osteoporosis in chronic conditions, such as rheumatoid arthritis, which require routine corticosteroids, especially when other risk factors are present, such as postmenopause and also in later life.[3–5]

Combination therapy

It is known that the bisphosphonates have to be given with calcium and vitamin D in order that optimum benefits may be obtained, otherwise no consideration to the study of therapeutic combination of treatments would have been given. Moreover there are limitations to the means of combining treatments because of the differences of the indications and modes of action.

One area in which combination therapy is an option is in post-menopausal women, as both HRT and bisphosphonates are indicated. A four-year study looked at etidronate and HRT both separately and in combination, in comparison with a calcium and vitamin D control group. Over the time period of the study, the combination therapy of etidronate and HRT showed the greatest improvement in bone mineral density at the hip and the spine.[12,13]

Side-effects

Only a few years into the first clinical trial of combination therapy, cases of osteomalacia were noted. This is a known complication of high-dose therapy in which the bone mass increase can actually undermine the bone strength. This remains a consideration in the long-term treatment with etidronate, due to the known bone mineralisation effect. Evidence of osteomalacia shows up as an increase in fractures.

The main side-effects originate, as with other bisphosphonates, in the gastrointestinal tract. They are nausea, abdominal pain, diarrhoea or constipation. Transient reduction in serum calcium and an increase in serum phosphate can occur; allergic skin reactions are also possible, causing itching, urticaria and angioedema. Headache, pins and needles, peripheral neuropathy are neurological effects; blood disorders such as agranulocytosis, leucopenia and pancytopenia are rarely reported.[8]

Risedronate

A recent introduction, this new bisphosphonate has characteristics similar to those of the other drugs within the group. Risedronate is administered at a dose of 5 mg every day for both the treatment and prevention of osteoporosis in postmenopausal women with or without corticosteroid-induced disease. It is given as a continuous regimen which requires that the patient has an adequate intake of calcium and vitamin D. If this is not the case then supplements must be given.

As with other bisphosphonates, risedronate has a low intestinal absorption of between 0.5 and 3%, therefore it is imperative that everything is done to enhance absorption. Advice on taking risedronate is as follows: it must be taken at least 30 minutes before consuming the first food of the day, alternatively no food should be consumed for two hours prior to taking or for two hours afterwards. This prevents the interaction with calcium-containing food, such as milk, iron, mineral supplements and antacid mixtures. To aid absorption and to prevent upper gastrointestinal irritation, it is advised that risedronate is taken with a reasonable volume of water, at least 120 ml. The large volume of water serves two purposes: it facilitates dissolution and it lubricates the passage of the tablets down the oesophagus. In order to reduce the possibility of upper gastrointestinal irritation, patients should be advised to take the drug whilst standing and not to lie down for a further 30 minutes after taking the medication.[8]

Clinical effectiveness

Risedronate has been evaluated in a number of clinical trials for both prevention and treatment of osteoporosis in postmenopausal women. The common end points of these trials are the increase in bone mass and the reduction in incidence of fracture rate. Risedronate has been shown to increase bone mass over the short term, that is a period of one or two years; similar benefits have been seen in the reduction of vertebral and hip fractures. The advantage that risedronate may have over other drugs is that the reduction in fracture rate is seen within the relatively short period of six months.

A large clinical study looked at women who were at least five years postmenopausal and had established osteoporosis, manifested in some as a low bone mineral density in the spine coupled with one vertebral fracture or in others as two vertebral fractures.[14] The patients received risedronate in association with calcium and vitamin D to ensure that they obtained the minimum requirements from these supplements and diet. In the first year of treatment there was a 65% reduction in the risk of vertebral fracture in comparison with the placebo control group. The reduction of risk continued throughout the trial period of three years, together with increases in bone mineral density at the spine and femoral neck of the hip. Similar work carried out on the use of risedronate to reduce the rate of hip fractures in older women aged 70–79 and over 80 showed a significant reduction in hip fractures.

Risedronate has also been used in one clinical trial in post-menopausal women who had corticosteroid-induced osteoporosis. Progress in these patients, who had been taking corticosteroids for at least 12 months prior to treatment, was studied over a period of one year. A significant increase in bone mineral density along with a reduction in fracture risk was shown.[14–16]

Side-effects

The risedronate side-effect profile shows similarities to the other bisphosphonates, in particular the risk of upper gastrointestinal problems. If the recommended method of administration is strictly adhered to then this will limit possible side-effects, but in patients with pre-existing or suffering from other oesophageal problems the therapy would need to be discontinued. Other gastrointestinal side-effects include abdominal pain, diarrhoea, constipation, nausea and colitis. Central nervous side-effects include headache and dizziness; respiratory problems include apnoea, bronchitis and sinusitis. Musculoskeletal side-effects such as bone pain and muscle pain are rarely seen. Other mild side-effects are skin rashes and effects on the eye and ear.

Other bisphosphonates

There are a number of other bisphosphonates available which are known to have similar effects on bone metabolism, but have not as yet been adopted as routine treatment for osteoporosis. Initially these drugs have been developed for the treatment of Paget's disease, a chronic condition of bone leading to deformities of the skeleton causing pain. Bisphosphonates are used to reduce the deformities and bone pain, but at much higher doses due to the degree of bone involvement. Whether a drug is evaluated for the treatment of osteoporosis or not depends on its success in treating Paget's disease. Two such drugs, which have shown some efficacy in osteoporosis, are clodronate and pamidronate, although these are restricted to the treatment of osteolytic lesions in patients suffering from cancer who have developed bone metastases. These drugs help to reduce bone pain and the associated hypercalcaemia of the malignant condition. Pamidronate, while effective in the treatment of osteoporosis, is limited by being available only as an injectable form in the UK. Clodronate, although available in an oral form and studied as a therapy for osteoporosis in either a continuous regimen or used every other month, has not been marketed for prevention or treatment.

A study of another bisphosphonate called tiludronate has provided evidence of efficacy in the treatment of osteoporosis, but a licence has not been obtained for use in either prevention or treatment. One other drug, ibandronate, has been used in studies in the form of either a daily oral treatment or a three-monthly injection, but further work is awaited to obtain proof of efficacy.

Comparison of bisphosphonates

To date there have been no comparative studies of two or more bisphosphonates in one clinical trial. In pharmacoeconomic studies, carried out based on previous individual drug trials, the comparisons drawn have been on the basis of the number of patients needed to be treated to prevent one fracture. A recent study comparing etidronate and risedronate, looked at the costs in preventing hip fracture in women. Although risedronate proved to be more cost effective, the number of suppositions and projections based on data for a three-year period limits the validity. Obviously a more direct comparison over a longer period would provide better analysis of the available data.[17]

References

1. *Martindale. The Extra Pharmacopoeia*, 28th edn. London: The Pharmaceutical Press 1982.
2. Kanis J A. *Osteoporosis*. Oxford: Blackwell Science, 1997.
3. Storm T, Thamsborg G, Steiniche T, *et al*. Effect of intermittent cyclical etidronate therapy on bone mass and fracture rate in women with postmenopausal osteoporosis. *N Engl J Med* 1990; **323**: 1265–1271.
4. Watts N B, Harris S T, Genant K, *et al*. Intermittent cyclical etidronate treatment of postmenopausal osteoporosis. *N Engl J Med* 1990; **323**: 73–79.
5. Harris S T, Watts N B, Jackson R D, *et al*. Four year study of etidronate treatment of postmenopausal osteoporosis. *Am J Med* 1993; **95**: 557–567.
6. Liberman U A, Weiss S R, Bröll J, *et al*. Effect of oral alendronate on bone mineral density and the incidence of fractures in postmenopausal osteoporosis. *N Engl J Med* 1995; **333**: 1437–1443.
7. Tonino R P, Meunier P J, Emkey R, *et al*. Skeletal benefits of alendronate: 7 year treatment of postmenopausal osteoporotic women. *J Clin Endocrinol Metab* 2000; **85**: 3109–3115.
8. *British National Formulary* No. 46. London: British Medical Association and Royal Pharmaceutical Society, 2003.
9. Orwoll E, Ettinger M, Weiss S, *et al*. Alendronate treatment of osteoporosis in men. *J Bone Miner Res* 1999; **14**(1 Suppl): S184.
10. Adachi J D, Bensen W G, Brown J, *et al*. Intermittent etidronate therapy to prevent corticosteroid-induced osteoporosis. *N Engl J Med* 1997; **337**: 382–387.
11. Levine M A H, Grootendorst P. Proportion of postmenopausal women at increased risk for upper GI adverse events associated with bisphosphonate therapy. *Pharmac Drug Saf* 2000; **9**: 367–370.
12. Wimalawansa S J. A four-year randomised control of hormone replacement and biphosphonate, alone and in combination in women with postmenopausal osteoporosis. *Am J Med* 1998; **104**: 219–226.
13. Ravn P, Bidstrup M, Wasnich R D, *et al*. Alendronate and estrogen-progestin in the long-term prevention of bone loss. *Ann Intern Med* 1999; **131**: 935–942.
14. McClung MR, Geusens P, Miller P, *et al*. Effect of risedronate on the risk of hip fracture in elderly women. *N Engl J Med* 2001; **344**: 333–340.
15. Reginster J Y, Minne H W, Sorensen O H, *et al*. Randomised trial of the effects of risedronate on vertebral fractures in women with established postmenopausal osteoporosis. *Osteoporosis Int* 2000; **11**: 83–91.
16. Harris S T, Watts N B, Genant H K, *et al*. Effects of risedronate treatment on vertebral and nonvertebral fractures in women with postmenopausal osteoporosis. *JAMA* 1999; **282**: 1344–1352.

17. Iglesias C, Torgerson D. Is risedronate more cost effective than etidronate for fracture prevention? A cost-utility analysis. *Proceedings of the Annual European Conference of the International Society of Pharmacoeconomics and Outcomes Research, Antwerp, Belgium,* 2000: 3.

11

The future

What does the future hold in store with regard to osteoporosis? Will the nature of the disease alter? Will the incidence in the population change? Will there be new remedies or treatments available to offer patients? These are some of the fundamental questions for which answers must be sought in order to know what the future has in store as far as the prevention and treatment of osteoporosis is concerned. To answer some of these questions it is necessary to analyse the current situation and see how it could possibly evolve in the next five to ten years, based on what we already know. What comparisons can be drawn from other similar conditions and are there developments in other fields that could be applied to osteoporosis?

Population demographics

We are currently aware that people in the Western world are living longer than ever before and enjoying a reasonable quality of life into old age. There are more people, within the population who are living to become octogenarians and older and this trend would appear likely to continue. If anything, experts predict that in the future people will be living a great deal longer and that life expectancy will continue to rise.

This increase in longevity is derived from a number of factors relating to overall improvements in public health. Elements include vaccination against common childhood illnesses, better nutrition, availability of free healthcare, education in and more awareness of good health practices, improved standard of living conditions, sanitation and housing. All these factors have increased the likelihood of surviving the normal childhood illnesses, eliminating fatal disease epidemics in adulthood and maintaining health through promotion to stave off chronic disease.

The net effect of this is that people are either avoiding disease or are contracting it much later in life, and once-fatal conditions can be either cured or ameliorated by medication. These advances have considerably reduced the number of fatal conditions and increased survival periods for others. A different spectrum of disease has developed, with patients' survival being controlled for many years on medication, often for more than one condition. Therefore, the well-being of the population lasting into later years is achieved by reducing the effects of wear and tear of the body, supplemented with adaptations either physical or chemical in the form of drug therapy.

The current elderly population of the UK grew up during a period of austerity, in the earlier part of the twentieth century, when life was harder than today and to survive through this period of economic depression followed by rationing, both during the war and for quite some time afterwards, was no mean feat. Life was very different then; both men and women were required to undertake more physical activity as part of the daily routine. This lifestyle, with a restriction in diet coupled with plenty of physical activity when at work and play meant that people who survived were in reasonable health, fit and able. This combination has been improved on in time with health promotion to reduce premature death by stopping smoking, reducing alcohol intake and increased exercise. The cohort of the population who are just about to enter their latter years have lived a more stable life, due to the general improvement in the quality of life through a better standard of living. The rise in the standard of living and the enhanced quality of life that ensued brought about an explosion in the UK birth rate in the 1950s and 1960s. Since then, the population and birth rate has decreased as people have gained more control over their lives and the way they live, maintaining a better quality of life for longer. All these contributing factors have led to an increased proportion of the adult population who live much beyond pensionable age and continue to be active well into later life. Therefore, the demographic changes have produced a population that is at increasing risk of osteoporosis if interventions are not encouraged.[1,2]

Lifestyle changes

There has been a gradual change in the lifestyle of people in Western countries, as compared with that of, say, 10 or 20 years ago. The main reason for this is that the quality and standard of life has improved; we are now more dependent on motorised transport, labour-saving devices are the norm, our eating habits have changed, the amount of physical activity we undertake is different, and levels of alcohol intake and smoking have altered radically. Let us explore the trends in each of these lifestyle factors and examine how these will affect the prevalence of osteoporosis.

Smoking

The level of smoking in the general population is decreasing in the UK; more and more people have given up smoking in adult life. Unfortunately, the number of teenagers who start smoking has remained more or less the same and there are just as many girls who smoke as boys. The trend is that there will be more girls than boys smoking in the future. This is bad news for the effect on the incidence of osteoporosis. Smoking has two main detrimental effects: first there is a direct effect on bone, reducing the optimum bone mass achieved; secondly, in women smoking reduces the protective action of oestrogen on maintaining bone mass. Therefore the overall response to the change in the picture of cigarette smoking is that there will be a lower peak bone mass achieved; but as people stop in later life the rate of bone loss will be reduced. This alteration in smoking habits will increase the incidence of osteoporosis in women more than in men due to the dual action of smoking on bone loss in women.

Alcohol

The consumption of alcohol in the UK is increasing as it becomes cheaper, relatively speaking, and is more aggressively marketed in different forms that appeal to young and old alike. Furthermore, the trend is towards younger and younger people drinking alcohol on a regular basis and increasingly drinking to excess. In the past, alcohol consumption had been highest among young men, but in the last ten years consumption by young women has been catching up rapidly, as it becomes a more acceptable facet of modern life.

Alcohol is available today in a much wider range of forms than previously; in the past there was only wine, beer, fortified drinks and spirits, but the introduction of 'alcopops', a mixture of soft drinks with varying amounts of spirits, has encouraged people to commence consumption of alcohol at an ever-younger age. A heavy-drinking culture has arisen among certain groups of young people, in which status is gained based on the amount they can consume or the strength of the alcoholic beverage with which they can cope. This culture conveys the message that it is good to consume large quantities of the strongest alcohol available.

The increase in alcohol consumption in the young will have a growing detrimental effect on their bone production, reducing their ability to attain the optimum bone mass. The legacy of this is that when bone loss starts later in adult life, it will be from a lower level, increasing the potential for osteoporosis and the consequential risk of fracture.

This is a particular hazard in women because of their lower optimum bone mass and because of the effect of the menopause.

Physical exercise

The amount of weight-bearing physical exercise an individual takes in their formative years will influence their ability to achieve a reasonable peak bone mass in early adult life. If physical exercise is continued into adult life, it will help to maintain bone mass and arrest the slow loss that starts after the peak bone mass is attained. The beneficial effects remain for only a short period once regular exercise has stopped; therefore, to maintain the advantage, exercise should be taken on a regular basis over a reasonable length of time.

During recent years, the level of exercise undertaken by the general population in the UK has declined, in particular by children who would gain the greatest benefit. This trend in children is a direct result of the gradual exclusion of competitive sport as part of the school curriculum at all levels of education. The growth in popularity in computer games and the increased use of computers by children means that many spend a great deal of their free time in sedentary occupation. This type of behaviour is increasingly carried on into adult life, when traditional sport is given up. With more and more employment requiring minimal physical effort, the opportunity for physical exercise is limited. The growth of certain sports, health clubs and gymnasiums has in a small way bucked the trend, but this has not been sufficient to encourage enough people to take up exercise on a regular basis.

If these trends continue and the population as a whole continues to follow a largely sedentary lifestyle, with little or no weight-bearing exercise, the risk of osteoporosis will increase.

In contrast to the risks associated with lack of exercise, it should be noted that too much exercise, especially in conbination with a low-calorie diet, can also be harmful to bone health. Some female athletes, especially long distance runners, find that they cease menstruating as a result of a combination of excessive exercise and a low body weight. This means that they lose the protective effect of the female sex hormones.

Diet

In order to ensure that development in the formative years follows a natural progression without any controls or hindrance to growth, the diet should be balanced and should contain all the essential nutrients, vitamins and minerals. In particular, in the avoidance of osteoporosis, the diet should contain adequate sources of calcium and vitamin D in order to promote the normal development of bone to peak bone mass. Any deficiencies of these vital vitamins and minerals will lead to a lower than predicted bone mass; in extreme situations deformities of the long bones will result.

In recent years, changes in the modern diet have led to the exclusion of a number of foods that were commonplace 20 or 30 years ago. Often these absent foods have been replaced with foods that are actually detrimental to development, as they not only contain less essential nutrients but also tend to flush out the valuable nutrients that are ingested. An example of this is the reduced intake of dairy products, which are rich in calcium and vitamin D and which have been replaced with carbonated drinks. Other trends include the increasing dependence on junk food, which has a high fat content, as opposed to a more balanced diet containing larger quantities of fruit and vegetables.

Eating disorders, which by their very nature lead to poor nutrition, can be disastrous for bone development. Anorexia nervosa, particularly in young women, has become a major problem. This is a disorder characterised by deliberate weight loss, sustained by the patient because she feels that she is too fat. In young women the effects on the body in general are compounded by the effect on menstruation, which ceases when the body weight falls below a critical level. The cessation of menstruation decelerates the loss of further essential nutrients, but it cannot compensate for the loss of the sex hormones required to prevent calcium loss from bone. Women with a long history of anorexia nervosa will be in danger of premature osteoporosis and fractures in early adult life rather than after the menopause.

The dietary changes mentioned above and the increasing prevalence of eating disorders both promote the early development of osteoporosis and both have a major impact on quality of life in later years. If a patient with a serious eating disorder survives into later adulthood, the likelihood of early death remains high following multiple fractures because of the development of osteoporosis.

Lifestyle trends

Taking all these changes in lifestyle factors into consideration – the trend towards increased alcohol intake, smoking at an earlier age, more sedentary lifestyles and failure to follow a healthily balanced diet – it is clear that we are heading towards a situation in which a large proportion of the population will be at greater risk of developing osteoporosis. Although there has been a noted decrease in the incidence of heart disease and certain cancers, which indicates that health promotion messages are making an impact, there needs to be even greater progress before the looked for reduction in osteoporotic fractures can be achieved.[3]

Health factors

The major contributing factor that indicates the likelihood of an individual developing osteoporosis is the genetic make-up. First, there are major differences in the sexes, with women four times more likely to suffer the consequences of osteoporosis than men. Women who have a family history of osteoporosis have a one in two chance of developing osteoporosis themselves. Currently the identification of these women at greatest risk is a matter of chance, or persistence by the individuals. Recent advances in gene technology, however, offer the prospect of the isolation of the relevant gene or genetic material, enabling the identification of those who will probably suffer from osteoporosis in later life. If a simple genetic test could be created to identify those people at risk of osteoporosis, then this would be a major advance. It would depend on the economics of the test as to whether it was employed as a screening test or used mainly as a research tool.

If it were possible to predict when women would enter the menopause and how quickly their sex hormone levels would fall then early preventative action might be taken. As discussed previously, the earlier the menopause and the faster the decline in oestrogen levels, the greater will be a woman's bone mass loss. This will forecast whether the woman will develop osteoporosis sooner rather than later and the likelihood of suffering the consequential fractures that can occur. If there was a method of identifying the timing of the menopause for each woman and then delaying that for as long as possible, would this be better than replacement therapy after the event? What would be the consequences of delaying the menopause? Would this be the same as replacement therapy, which delays the progression to osteoporosis? Hormone replacement therapy (HRT) is known to increase the risk of breast cancer and of heart disease; these adverse effects could perhaps be eliminated by inducing the female body to continue to produce the sex hormones instead of administering synthetic hormone. Research into the use of stem cells is being carried out to discover whether they could be implanted into various organs or sites to regenerate tissue and to maintain the required level of the sex hormones.[4]

Monitoring

The initial diagnosis and ongoing monitoring of osteoporosis relies on access to a dual-energy X-ray absorptiometry (DEXA) scanner, which measures the density of bone either at particular points of the skeleton or of the whole body. Lack of access to these scanners restricts the potential for diagnosis and there are a large number of hospitals in the UK that do not possess a scanner. Even if a hospital does possess a DEXA scanner then the high demand for use and the limited available time ensures that waiting lists for scans extend into months. The result of this restricted use is that only those patients whose diagnosis is more than likely to prove positive will be allocated a scan. Others, who are not seen as being at clinical risk, are discouraged from having a scan due to long waiting times. This means that strict criteria are required to identify those patients in the greatest need of diagnosis and monitoring with these scanners. The robust management of access is a necessary requirement for the most effective use of the scanner in order to obtain the most efficient number of positive results from the patients treated.

Until there is a vast increase in the number of available DEXA scanners in the UK, together with the skilled operators who are required to carry out the tests and the interpretation of the results, then there will always be a problem in making an early diagnosis and having the ability to monitor the effectiveness of treatment. For the future, access to the scanners should be readily available for those patients known to be at risk of osteoporosis because of family history, early menopause or corticosteroid usage. Not only would this provision be a minimum requirement in identifying those people at greatest risk, but it would also provide the ability to monitor those patients who are being treated for osteoporosis and to screen people who are at risk because of lifestyle factors.

The use of DEXA scanners in the very earliest stages at the commencement of the progression to osteoporosis would pinpoint those people requiring intervention with active treatment, in order to prevent a deterioration in their quality of life. The longer osteoporosis is allowed to develop without treatment to reduce or arrest bone mass loss, the more likely a fracture is to occur with the possibility of a detrimental effect on the quality of life. Once treatment is initiated, if monitoring is not completed on an annual basis, then the effectiveness of the medication is unknown, particularly if the chosen drug is no longer capable of reversing the bone mass loss.

The major disadvantages of using a DEXA scanner to diagnose and monitor bone mass loss is that the scanner is expensive both to buy and to operate. The economics of use is the limiting factor on the availability. If there were a simple cheap test, which allowed for ease of use by non-skilled operators, then availability would increase. Diagnosis at the moment relies on imaging of the bone and measuring the density, and if this could be executed in a simpler more cost effective manner, using an alternative imaging system then it would be adopted. If a factor or biochemical substance could be isolated and tested using a dipstick for urine or blood, then this would make a significant difference, as has been witnessed in other chronic conditions.[5]

Medical interventions

Although surgical interventions to repair fractures caused by osteoporosis can improve mobility in the short term and great advances in the design and use of prostheses have been made, the condition of the bone at this stage is poor and the results are never ideal in the long term. This type of surgery is very invasive; most operations to repair fractures take over an hour to complete and are associated with a number of complications. If it is apparent that the state of the bone is such that another fracture may occur at any time, then the surgical option will only be embarked upon as a last resort. This makes the success rate all the more remarkable. Neverthless, great improvements could be made with the development of less invasive surgery, which causes minimal trauma to the bone, and the production of a new type of prosthesis that is easier to attach and that does not react with surrounding tissue.

Many different drugs are used in the treatment and prevention of osteoporosis, dependent on the stage of the condition and whether the patient is male or female. The following section discusses the current treatments used and how they may be developed in the future.[6]

Calcium

Supplements of calcium have been used in both the treatment and prevention of osteoporosis. The dose of calcium needed as a supplement has been studied extensively, taking into consideration the normal dietary intake. Calcium supplements have been notoriously difficult to formulate into a palatable preparation that patients are willing to take on a regular basis. There are now a few chewable calcium tablets, soluble tablets and granular formulations that are relatively pleasant to take. Adequate calcium intake will always be necessary to help to replace the bone mass lost in osteoporosis, but there is little to be gained from the continued use of calcium unless combination preparations with other drugs, for example the bisphosphonates, are considered.

Vitamin D

The use of vitamin D in its different forms as an adjunct treatment in osteoporosis, usually in combination with calcium, has been researched in depth. This has led to the recommendation of an ideal dosage of vitamin D to be used in conjunction with calcium and the formulation as a combination product with calcium. The further development of vitamin D preparations is unlikely as all the possible analogues have been tried and there is too little difference between them to justify more research. Following clinical studies there have been a number of calcium and vitamin D combination preparations used as standard treatment as an adjunct to either HRT or bisphosphonates. The most likely development in this area is a combination preparation of calcium and vitamin D with a bisphosphonate either as a pack with separate tablets or as one tablet containing the three ingredients. The latter option is less likely unless a bisphosphonate can be found that does not interact with calcium to reduce absorption.

Hormone replacement therapy

There have been a number of advances in the use and presentation of HRT since the introduction of the first oestrogen tablets, indicated for women who had undergone a premature surgical menopause. At the time, this was thought to be the only requirement for usage. It was not until women started to demand a remedy for the symptoms associated with the process of going through the menopause that other indications and medications were researched. Today, we have a variety of preparations, including continuous oestrogen, continuous oestrogen with opposing intermittent progestogen and continuous oestrogen with continuous progestogen. In addition, the administration of these hormones can now be presented in a variety of different pharmaceutical forms, ranging from the usual tablets in various calendar packs to topical patches containing the hormone for use at up to seven-day intervals. The next step would be to develop longer lasting treatment options; these hormone preparations exist now, but as a long-acting contraceptive. There is no reason why, with the manipulation of the hormonal content, the depot presentations in the form of subcutaneous matrix rods, deep intramuscular depot injections and intrauterine devices presently used

MANAGEMENT FOCUS

Improved selectivity and formulation of medications to aid patient acceptability and compliance

Hormone replacement therapy – available in long-term depot devices, more selective, reduced cardiac side-effects

Bisphosphonates – availability of long-acting injectable forms

for contraception could not be used for HRT. These preparations can deliver sex hormones for up to five years, which is ideal for the two main uses of hormone replacement therapy: the relief of postmenopausal symptoms and the long-term prevention of osteoporosis. Depot formulations would improve patient compliance over the required period and would reduce the total content of sex hormones delivered, thus minimising side-effects (see Management Focus, above).

HRT, which has the potential to be given for a period of up to 20 years, shows an inconsistent uptake amongst postmenopausal women. Despite all the detailed research into the use of HRT, there are still questions with regard to the ideal length of treatment. Initially HRT was given continuously for as long as the patients were willing to tolerate and comply with the regimen. Often, after only a few years, symptom control of the menopause was achieved and patients became unwilling to continue taking the HRT. However, clinical trials have shown that a treatment period of at least seven years is required to reduce the detrimental effects of osteoporosis. Because the use of HRT for longer than 5–10 years can lead to some long-term adverse effects, it has been proposed that a more appropriate method of use would be to restrict it to a 2–3 year period around the menopause and to restart the therapy some time later for a much longer time, in order to prevent osteoporosis. This manipulation would not be necessary if the long-term risks, such as breast cancer and thromboembolic conditions, could be reduced.[7,8]

The next development was the discovery of the selective oestrogen receptor modulator (SERM) drugs, which reduce the incidence of breast cancer in women who have been prescribed HRT. Raloxifene, the first drug in this group to be launched, was quickly followed by other drugs with a similar action. At first this was a theoretical consideration, as the SERM drugs do not act on the oestrogen receptors found in the breast. After further clinical trials SERM drugs have proved effective in the short term of a few years. These benefits have been identified initially for women who have either a family history of breast cancer or a previously diagnosed disease.

Another adverse effect of HRT is the detrimental effect on pre-existing cardiac disease and the precipitation of heart disease in treated women. Initially, HRT was thought to be beneficial in preventing cardiac disease, as premenopausal women have a much lower incidence of cardiac disease than men of the same age. Unfortunately, after a number of clinical studies there have been many conflicting reports, some stressing the benefits and others emphasising the harmful effects. Recently, the UK Committee on Safety of Medicines directed that HRT should not be prescribed for the prevention of cardiac disease and that it should be stopped if coronary heart disease develops. Clearly, if a HRT could be found that is as effective in preventing heart disease as SERM drugs are in preventing breast cancer, this could be used for long-term therapy in patients with a pre-existing cardiac disease.[9–11]

Bisphosphonates

The development of an oral form of bisphosphonate was a major advance and led to the use of these drugs in the treatment and prevention of osteoporosis. The main problem with all these drugs is that they are poorly absorbed from the gastrointestinal tract and that they interact with food, thus reducing the absorption. Even given ideal conditions, absorption is only 5–15% of the oral dose, which limits the efficacy of the drug. The other problem with all bisphosphonates to a lesser or greater extent is the adverse effect of irritation on the upper gastrointestinal tract. This can be lessened by taking the medication with a large volume of water and then not lying down for at least 30 minutes.

Researchers have approached these problems in different ways. One method has been to formulate a tablet to be taken once per week rather than once per day. This ensures that the patient only has to tolerate possible side-effects once a week rather than every day. Also, the effort required to get up early to take the medication before breakfast and remain upright for 30 minutes afterwards is lessened. The other option is to formulate an injection to be given every three months. However, the two drugs that are available for this purpose as injections are not yet indicated for either prevention or treatment of osteoporosis, although clinical trials have shown that they have efficacy. Presently under clinical evaluation is an annual injection of zoledronic acid, which has been shown to raise bone density at the spine and hip. The use of zoledronic acid produces effects similar to those of the shorter acting drugs, but it has the advantage that the dose is given as a 15-minute infusion whereas with the other drugs the infusion spans a number of hours. The use of zoledronic acid would seem to be a major advance in bisphosphonate therapy if the initial potential can be carried through to a long-term therapy. The outstanding unknown factor is the acceptability to patients of this short duration infusion, even though it would be just once a year.[12]

Other drugs

Fluoride has been the subject of a number of clinical studies, but it has failed to give consistently good results in the long term. The bone produced under the influence of fluoride was not of the same strength as the existing bone and the use of fluoride could lead to a weakening of the bones. A recently developed drug that has shown some promising results is strontium ranelate, which is currently undergoing clinical trials in phase III studies in postmenopausal women. This strontium derivative has been shown to increase bone formation and to reduce bone absorption, but only time will tell if this continues to show potential in reducing fractures over a long period.[13]

Health promotion

There has been no national campaign of health promotion in the UK to highlight the problems of osteoporosis that can occur in later life. This may be due to the fact that, unlike heart disease or cancer, osteoporosis does not have such a dramatic life or death effect. When the level of morbidity and the economic considerations of treatment are realised, then we may get the political will to do something about the causes of the condition. The messages to get across for the prevention of osteoporosis are the same as those for a number of conditions – to avoid the usual evils of smoking, consumption of excess alcohol and the lack of exercise.

Osteoporosis is a condition of the elderly, who are currently not economically viable. However, the increase in the elderly population and the cost to the nation of ongoing treatment should soon awaken interest in prevention. At the moment any campaigning to create awareness is through the patients' association, who do a good job but who are not able to resource large-scale national advertising. Hopefully in the future this will be resourced properly, giving a chance for the message to get through to those within the population who are at greatest risk.[2]

Health screening

At present there is no national health screening policy for osteoporosis in the UK. There are some local schemes, which are dependent on a local initiative originating from an interested party. This type of service can be disjointed and sometimes fails to link up a number of services to allow the identification of the people at greatest risk. Often, only those who become aware of this service through word of mouth can benefit. The lack of information limits the effectiveness of the service to the majority of the population. Resources at present are not based on known requirements, but are there as an add-on function to an existing service.

The National Osteoporosis Society (NOS) and the Royal College of Physicians have developed guidelines for screening, but these have not been taken up at a national level nor funded centrally, with targets of number of patients seen and treated. There are no incentives for doctors to identify those patients at risk, in fact there is a disincentive in the form of additional drug costs. The active mechanisms for ensuring minimum standards of care are the National Service Frameworks (NSF), which have been created to oversee several groups of illnesses. These NSFs set out in detail service levels and targets that need to be met by a set time period, which encourages both clinical audit and research into the effectiveness of the guidance. If an NSF were adopted for osteoporosis, this would stimulate the production of an integrated national service.[1]

Fall prevention

Although fracture prevention either by maintaining bone mass or by reducing bone loss is seen as the ultimate outcome of osteoporosis treatment, these fractures could be prevented by avoiding the falls that usually cause them. Falls often result in a fractured neck of the femur or colles fracture. If it is possible to prevent such a fall happening in the first place, then this will show a parallel reduction in the incidence of fractures. There are a number of reasons for a fall, including drug-induced drowsiness, diminished physical ability in walking due to frailty and the hazards that exist in everyday life. These reasons can all be examined and ways in which to reduce the risk addressed.

Much research has been carried out into the use of benzodiazepines – particularly administration in the elderly – for night sedation and the consequential after-effects on the following day. This has provoked the movement away from long-acting drugs such as nitrazepam, the after-effects of which can last for up to 18 hours. Even the shorter acting benzodiazepines are found to have a long duration of action in the elderly, who, because of their reduced liver function, take longer to metabolise the drug. The newer agents, the imidazopyridine derivatives, although unrelated to benzodiazepines, appear to possess the same characteristics, causing the next-day drowsiness and dizziness. Guidelines have been drawn up to reduce the use of these drugs, especially in the elderly; if they are used, the length of course should be held to a maximum of seven days. There is still, however, widespread use of these drugs as a result of public demand and because it is known that withdrawal symptoms probably occur on discontinuing treatment. These drugs are not completely safe in the elderly and should be avoided if at all possible. Public education programmes to promote the view that as you get older there is less need for sleep could be effective in reducing demand.

Various studies have attempted to analyse the environmental risks posed to the elderly, in order to minimise the risk of falling. In one such study, modifications were made to the homes of a group of elderly persons and the number of subsequent falls over a 12-month period was compared with that in a control group, where visits were made only for social or health reasons. Although the results showed a significant reduction in the number of falls, there was no corresponding reduction in the number of fractures. This suggests that the ability to modify risk is not sufficient and other factors must be reviewed before the incidence of fractures is decreased together with the number of falls.[14]

Another approach centred on an attempt to reduce the impact of any fall and thus decrease the incidence of fractures with protective padding. One study investigating the use of hip protectors in elderly residents in nursing homes, used external padded hip protectors incorporated into special underwear. One group of residents were given the hip protectors and the control group were not. The result was a 50% reduction in hip fractures in the protector group, and the only people in

MANAGEMENT FOCUS

How to improve management of osteoporosis
Health promotion – target different sections of the population with relevant information about osteoporosis, using all types of media
Health screening – introduce a programme, available through various health providers, aimed at those sections of the population most at risk
Fall prevention – inform health professionals of advice to be given to those at risk, set up clinics or help centres with relevant information

the protector group who did have a hip fracture were not wearing the protectors at the time. However, these hip protectors were found to be bulky and uncomfortable to wear. Clearly, if these aids are to be brought into common use in the future, such problems will have to be solved (see Management Focus, above).[15]

References

1. Royal College of Physicians. *Osteoporosis. Clinical Guidelines for Prevention and Treatment. Update on pharmacological interventions and an algorithm for management.* London: Royal College of Physicians, 2003.
2. International Osteoporosis Foundation. *Osteoporosis in the Workplace.* Liege, Belgium: WHO Collaborative Center, 2003.
3. Dinsdale P. Waking up to osteoporosis. *Health and Ageing* October 2000: 49.
4. National Osteoporosis Society. An osteoporosis framework – meeting health needs. www.nos.org.uk (accessed 2000).
5. Courtney A, Thomson F C, Watson A M, *et al.* Primary care implementation of specialist treatment recommendations for osteoporosis following hospital consultation for risk assess/DEXA scanning. *Pharmacy World and Science* 2002; **24**: A39–A40.
6. National Service Framework (NSF). *Older People.* London: Department of Health, 2001: Standard six: 76–89.
7. Rees M, Purdie D W. *Management of the Menopause: the Handbook of the British Menopause Society.* London: BMS Publications, 2002.
8. Papaioannou A, Parkinson W, Adachi J, *et al.* Women's decision about hormone replacement therapy after education and bone densitometry. *CMAJ* 1998; **159**: 1253–1257.
9. Rexrode K M, Manson J E. Postmenopausal hormone therapy and quality of life. *JAMA* 2002; **287**: 641–642.
10. Committee on Safety of Medicines. Safety update on long-term HRT. *Curr Probl Pharmacovigilance* 2002; **28**: 11–12.
11. Barrett-Connor E, Grady B, Sashegyi A, *et al.* Raloxifene and cardiovascular events in osteoporotic postmenopausal women. *JAMA* 2002; **287**: 847–857.
12. Cada D J, Levien T, Baker D. Zoledronic acid for injection. *Hosp Pharm* 2001; **36**: 1–8.
13. Meunier P. Novel osteoporosis treatment reduces incidence of new vertebral fractures. *Pharm J* 2002; **268**: 756.
14. Stott P. Don't fail older fallers. *Health and Ageing* February 2002: 30–32.
15. Parker M J, Gillespie L D, Gillespie W J. Hip protectors for preventing falls in the elderly (Cochrane Review). *The Cochrane Library* 2002, issue 4.

12

Osteoporosis screening

Whether or not the application of health screening is appropriate for a particular disease is dependent on a number of factors. The overriding consideration has to be whether the screening will identify, with near perfect accuracy, the early stages of the disease. If this is known, the case for introduction has to be argued on the basis of the cost of the screening programme against the likely cost saving that will ensue with improved quality in patients' lives. National breast and cervical cancer screening programmes currently running in the UK have been shown to result in a reduced mortality rate for these diseases. At present, researchers are attempting to develop a screening programme for coronary heart disease in order to reduce premature deaths from this condition.

The advantage of a national scheme of screening for a particular condition is that services are developed at the same rate across the country, giving an equal opportunity of identifying the condition. This is based on a standard procedure in the screening process, a minimum requirement for resources based on the size of the population served, linking of services across primary and secondary care and uniform thresholds for the treatment of the condition. To ensure that these benefits are obtained there is a need for an independent means of auditing the programme, in order to maintain uniform working standards of implementation, identification and treatment.

How does a national screening programme for osteoporosis in the UK fit into this pattern? First, it is worth reviewing the facts. There are clear known risk factors, which were first considered in the Department of Health Advisory Group Report on osteoporosis published in 1994,[1] and then developed further into a strategy for osteoporosis published four years later.[2] A part of this strategy was the production of guidelines by the Royal College of Physicians on the prevention and the treatment of the condition; these guidelines have since been updated to include an algorithm for management and treatments available.[3] It was further suggested that these guidelines should be developed in order that they may be endorsed by a number of other related Royal Colleges to promote awareness amongst other medical specialists. Thus, the ground-work has been completed for the introduction of a screening programme in the UK, but the organisation, implementation and management has been left to local health bodies, with the result that the service is sketchy, with no working model set up either as ideal or standard which could be promoted nationally.

There are two main approaches to health screening: the first is a catchall situation, whereby everybody goes through the screening process. This is used when there is no clear means of identifying those at greatest risk or those having the early indications of the disease. For this type of health screening, the test has to be inexpensive and must accurately predict the likelihood of the condition and offer a good chance of a complete cure following treatment. Early identification of the disease is beneficial as it permits treatment to have a significant effect on the outcome, as compared with the lesser benefits conferred when medication is commenced at a much later stage of the disease's progress. Examples of this type of disease are testicular and cervical cancer; if left to progress, these will lead to death, but if treated prior to spreading to other tissue then a complete cure is possible in the majority of cases.

An alternative method of identifying the section of the population at greatest risk of contracting a disease is based on enumerating the risk factors and assessing the degree to which the disease is present. This pro-cedure is used when a national screening programme fails to identify the disease or to pinpoint the incidence of subsequent outcomes suffered by individuals. The assessment of those felt to be most vulnerable should take the form of a simple questionnaire to which the answer should be either 'Yes' or 'No', rather than a scale of risk. Such a test should be undertaken prior to a more detailed pathological or diagnostic test, thus reducing the likelihood of producing negative results.

The use of a screening process will depend on the aim of the pro-gramme. In the case of osteoporosis, the prime objective is the preven-tion of fractures of the spine, hip or wrist. The timescale to the stage at which a fracture occurs can be a number of years; once a fracture has occurred the risk of a second is doubled. Therefore, if an assessment is left until a fracture is either highly likely, or has already taken place, the value is greatly diminished since the prospect of another fracture is more certain. Thus, the scale of any intervention is limited, in view of the certainty that a second fracture is inevitable because the bone mineral density is significantly low. By the time a fracture has occurred, the disease has progressed to a point at which the need for a bone mineral density measurement is eliminated, as treatment is a necessity.

To be of any merit, a screening test would have to be carried out during the initial stages of the disease, when the first signs of the condition can be identified, thus allowing an intervention to have a significant effect. To optimise the screening programme by identifying those at greatest risk, it is necessary to discover the ideal age, stage of life or contributing factor that will ensure that clinical intervention produces maximal effect. This leads to the selection of cohorts of the population that are high-risk groups; these people are required to be identified within the general health scheme to limit the detrimental effect of the disease. This should occur as part of a system of general health checks aimed at certain stages of life, where particular diseases are known to be prevalent, at a point at which an intervention will make a significant difference to health outcome. Osteoporosis is no different, in having a definite time of life when its presence becomes apparent, associated with particular life events, such as a family history as well as lifestyle habits and presence of specific diseases.[3,4]

At-risk groups

It is clearly necessary to identify the 'at-risk groups' for osteoporosis in order to catch the early stages of the disease when further investigation will be warranted. In the case of osteoporosis, the people considered to belong to the at-risk groups would meet the criteria listed in the Risk Factor Focus below.

RISK FACTOR FOCUS

Risk factors for osteoporosis
Parents with osteoporosis
Aged over 45
Postmenopausal women
Women with a premature menopause
Certain underlying diseases, e.g. chronic liver or renal disease
Certain drug regimens, e.g. long-term corticosteroids
Diet low in calcium and vitamin D
Lifestyle factors

A study of these at-risk groups is necessary to clarify the reasons for the risk factors and to explain why people at risk need further investigation with the aim of offering a definitive diagnostic test and optimal treatment to arrest the condition.[3-5]

Inherited osteoporosis

There is a strong association between genetic make-up and the risk of contracting osteoporosis. Inherited characteristics that are predictors of osteoporosis include female gender, white race and having a mother who has experienced a fracture due to lack of bone strength. These factors are important and identification of these will quickly highlight those women who are at the greatest risk, as has been confirmed from population studies that have audited people with the highest incidence of osteoporosis.

The basis of these predictors stems from the knowledge that an individual's optimum bone mass will be largely based on what his or her parents have achieved. This has both genetic and environmental factors: if the parents have participated in plenty of weight-bearing exercise, for example, then the offspring may well have been encouraged to do likewise. The maximum bone mass achieved and the manner in which it declines throughout the ageing process is defined largely by gender. In men, the maximum bone mass achieved is higher than in women, peaks around the mid-twenties, then declines slowly; in women the maximum reached is at a lower level and while the initial rate of decline is similar, once the menopause is reached, the rate of loss accelerates rapidly. This in itself shows that women are at greater risk of osteoporosis because of the lower bone mass and the way in which further bone loss occurs.

On average, women of white race are at greater risk of osteoporosis than women of other races; this is due to several factors related to lifestyle, their development, lack of physical activity, the span of the menstruation period, the number of children per family, the age at which the menopause commences and life expectancy. All these elements contribute to a greater risk of osteoporosis in white women than women of other races. Black and Asian women who move to Western countries and adopt a Western lifestyle display the same risk tendencies as white women.

The most compelling factor in predicting the likelihood of a person developing osteoporosis is whether or not their parents had the condition – particularly in their middle ages – more so if no other known risk factors prevail. All women whose mothers have had osteoporosis are at such high risk that, as they themselves enter the menopause, they should undergo screening as a matter of course. Such women are probably the most sensitive to the loss of female sex hormones, rapidly lose bone mass and very soon reach the stage where the extent of bone loss can easily precipitate a fracture. For such individuals, not only is screening at the onset of the menopause necessary, but they also require the beneficial effects of preventative treatment such as HRT.

Men in similar circumstances do not fare much better because, while not undergoing a process equivalent to the menopause, they still experience rapid loss of bone mass. Furthermore, men may experience a greater detrimental effect on their health because the condition may be allowed to progress to some extent before a diagnosis is considered. In men, the first sign of osteoporosis is often a loss in height due to vertebral compression fractures of the spine, at which stage preventative treatment is too late.

Age over 45

Once the age of 45 has been reached, both men and women will be losing bone mass and could well have reached a point at which the bone loss is both evident and predictive of the first signs of osteoporosis. For women, it is often the early stages of the menopause that is the most critical life event and that will determine if they will go on to suffer the consequences of osteoporosis. Once a woman has already passed through a natural menopause, then bone mass loss could be at the point where active treatment is necessary to reverse it. At the age of 45, most women will be about to enter the first stages of the menopause, which involves a rapid decline in the level of oestrogen release. At this stage, consideration should be given to preventative supplementary therapy. The process of the menopause can continue for a number of years and preventative treatment such as HRT may be chosen for the reduction of symptoms, rather than the more long-term condition of osteoporosis. Women are generally self-selecting according to their attitude, choosing when to come forward for preventative replacement therapy depending on the number and severity of the menopausal symptoms that they experience.

Men, on the other hand, do not undergo a similar stage in life, despite the speculation in the media as to the presence or absence of a 'male menopause', which is based on social trends rather than any physiological process. The level of male hormones does decline gradually over time, but no rapid loss occurs and there is not the same connection between loss of sex hormones and bone loss. Men who are at risk of osteoporosis may start to show signs of bone loss at this stage in their life, but it is only if other criteria are present that this would warrant further investigation.

Postmenopausal women

As stated earlier, the effect that the menopause has on a woman's long-term health is critical to the development of osteoporosis and her subsequent susceptibility to fractures in later life. As a risk factor for osteoporosis, menopausal status alone would not necessitate that every postmenopausal woman be screened, but consideration should be given to administering HRT in order to prevent bone loss. Where other related risk factors are present in a postmenopausal woman, further investigation is indicated, as the combination of certain risk factors could be highly indicative of the presence of osteoporosis.

Premature menopause

Menopause occurring prior to the age of 40 is defined as premature menopause. This condition results in a lack of oestrogen and the consequential loss of bone mass, leading to the onset of osteoporosis and increased risk of fractures. Ongoing quality of life may be affected and it may lead to an early death due to complications of further fractures, particularly of the spine and hip.

If a woman has a surgically induced premature menopause caused by removal of the uterus and ovaries as part of a hysterectomy operation, usually performed to treat cancer of the uterus or to remove fibroids, then replacement oestrogen therapy is given as a matter of course. This is in order to prevent the long-term effects of oestrogen deficiency and to alleviate the short-term symptoms, which are often self-limiting.

Certain underlying diseases

There are a number of diseases that have either a direct effect or an indirect effect on the ability of the body not only to form new bone but to maintain bone mass. In the main, these conditions restrict the availability of the required nutrients necessary for the manufacture of bone, namely calcium and vitamin D.

The reduced absorption of calcium or vitamin D caused by diseases of the gastrointestinal tract limit the ability of bone to achieve optimum mass during the development years. If a gastrointestinal condition is chronic and cannot be rectified to improve absorption up to normal levels, then osteoporosis will develop prematurely because of the persistently subnormal intake of calcium and vitamin D.

Chronic liver and renal disease will affect the body's ability to metabolise vitamin D to its active metabolites, which will reduce absorption of calcium and thus reduce bone formation, with the consequent increase in bone mass loss. In chronic renal failure this is a well-documented problem and supplements are given in the form of the activated form of vitamin D; however, in liver disease where the condition can be insidious it has only recently been recognised that supplementation with both calcium and vitamin D is a necessary requirement for these patients.

Conditions of the thyroid and parathyroid gland will affect the body's control over calcium balance, leading to hypo- or hypercalcaemia, both of which will affect bone development and bone strength. In hypercalcaemia there is overdepositing of calcium in the bone from stimulation of osteoclasts increasing bone resorption, resulting in osteolytic lesions with or without osteopenia. Hypocalcaemia will lead to poor bone development and structure; the bones formed will have a low bone mass with inadequate strength, leading to the formation of brittle bones, which are easily fractured following low-impact injuries.

Drug-induced osteoporosis

Anion-exchange resins, such as colestyramine, affect the absorption of vitamin D by chelation of the vitamin onto the resin, rendering the vitamin unavailable for absorption in the normal way. This effect only causes problems in elderly patients receiving chronic therapy, in whom the effects of therapy and age coexisting together increase the risk of osteoporosis and subsequent fracture.

Levothyroxine (thyroxine) has also been associated with osteoporosis, but it has not been established whether this was the side-effect of any previous thyrotoxicosis or caused solely by the drug. Obviously if a patient is given levothyroxine which leads to thyrotoxicosis, then this will increase the risk of osteoporosis, but even in chronic therapy when only sufficient levothyroxine is given to maintain thyroid function there is a small risk of osteoporosis.

The group of drugs that has the greatest potential to cause osteoporosis is the corticosteroids, particularly when given at a high dose, that is the equivalent of 7.5 mg or more of prednisolone over a number of months. The use of corticosteroids in this way leads to a rapid demineralisation of bone within a period of three to six months. If a high-dose regimen is indicated, then there will be a strong likelihood of the presence of osteoporosis within the first few months. Even the long-term use of lower doses of corticosteroids induces a degree of bone mineralisation, due to the cumulative effect of the presence of the drug.

Diet low in calcium and vitamin D

Vitamin D is necessary for the absorption and regulation of calcium uptake from the diet and its use within the body, particularly with relevance to use within the bone. It follows, therefore, that a reduction in vitamin D will have an automatic consequential effect on calcium, leading to hypocalcaemia. Vitamin D is only present in a few vital foods and the main source is from the effect of sunlight on the skin. If a person is on a self-induced exclusion diet, or is not exposed to enough sunlight throughout the year, there is a high probability of vitamin D deficiency.

Calcium is readily available from dairy products, but a reduced intake of these foods by people of all ages can easily result in lack of calcium. Many people have excluded either milk or cheese voluntarily from their daily food or have substituted low-calcium content foods in place of these dairy products because of a fear of allergy.

Lifestyle factors

The usual advice issued to people about lifestyle practices that can give rise to osteoporosis is to stop smoking and reduce the intake of alcohol, both of which have a seriously harmful effect on bone formation. Emphasis can also be given to the benefits of following an adequately nutritional diet rich in calcium and vitamin D, and of participation in weight-bearing exercise to establish and maintain a high bone mass.

Identifying patients at risk

Once the criteria necessary to identify patients at risk have been established, the next step should be to draw up a health questionnaire to be directed at those sections of the population deemed most likely to be at risk. The process of selecting and targeting these people will need some thought. Are they likely to be pre-existing patients attending a hospital, clinic or health professional for advice or treatment in respect of other health problems? Should people be approached through a general health awareness programme such as a Well Woman or Well Man Clinic set up within a GP's surgery. In a recent instance, people visiting their local community pharmacist were screened to discover whether or not they were at risk of osteoporosis. All these options can be used, and in order to ensure that as many people as possible are identified, the net must be spread as widely as possible to cover a multitude of avenues: it is not enough to rely on people coming forward requesting further information and investigation.

The general health strategy of the nation should contain a section dealing with osteoporosis in order to give the general public more information on bone health and what measures they should take to improve it. This would increase awareness of osteoporosis amongst the population, enabling them to decide whether they require advice or referral to a health agency. The next step would be to build a framework for categorising and dealing with people, establishing whether they require further advice or referral for investigation or treatment.

For such a project to succeed, there is a requirement for a collaborative approach, involving all the health agencies, including one-stop health advice shops, primary care, community care, secondary care and social services. Within each of these health agencies, there is a body or individual who makes a decision regarding the ongoing care of the patient in relationship to the strategy of treatment and prevention. This should be reviewed on a regular basis to ensure compliance with national guidance from respected health bodies. National guidelines may have to be adapted to fit in with local needs and resources, based on the perception of the interested parties, from each of the health agencies. If this is a new service, then promotion through the local media will help to raise awareness and interest from the local population and encourage the people at risk to come forward.[6–8]

Clinical management

In order to aid the clinical management of osteoporosis, it is necessary to agree a programme that defines each stage of the disease and the type of patient who will fall into these categories. This will ensure a uniform approach and speed patients through the system, to enable the correct level of clinical care to be given for either treatment or prevention. The level of care will depend on the risk factors present, the age of the patient and the probability of a fracture occurring. The major clinical intervention at this stage would be referral for bone density measurement by means of a dual-energy X-ray absorptiometry (DEXA) scanner. This should be reserved for high-risk patients for whom the best form of treatment is undecided. The choice of clinical management must be defined for optimal care, not only in respect of drug therapy, but also for the avoidance of a fracture from normal daily activities.

In a clinical management programme, which practitioners are authorised to refer which patients and to whom should be clearly defined: this will ensure that there is the optimum use of resources. Patients who should be referred for further investigation include those with a family history of osteoporosis, those with previous low trauma fracture, those who have been using corticosteroids at a dosage in excess of physiological level for more than three months, and women in whom the menopause has occurred before 45 years of age and secondary to a predisposing condition. In these cases, it is necessary to measure bone density in order to establish the level of bone mass loss and to determine the consequent need for treatment or whether preventative measures would suffice. The exception to this would be the women with a menopause prior to the age of 45; these women should receive HRT as a matter of course, but if this preventative therapy is contraindicated then assessment for alternative treatment options will be necessary.

The assessment of bone mass loss should indicate what action should be taken thereafter: this should be standardised so that everyone within a defined range would get the same care, advice and access to treatment. The range of clinical interventions will vary from advice on lifestyle measures to active treatment, in combination with symptomatic relief for associated symptoms.

The standardisation of recommended treatments at the various stages of osteoporosis is essential in order to obtain an optimum improvement in the quality of life for the maximum number of patients. There will need to be some variation around a general theme; for instance, a small number of different pharmaceutical forms of HRT will be necessary to enable most women to comply with the medication. A definitive protocol of treatment options is required to enable patients to receive the same standards of care independent of whom they consult, whether GP or specialist consultant. This should be based on nationally agreed guidelines, taken from the best clinical evidence from evaluated clinical studies of treatment options.

In order to introduce effective preventative measures for osteoporosis, it is necessary to target at-risk groups at the earliest possible moment and make these patients aware of the possibility of osteoporosis. This should be followed by further advice on ways of avoiding the consequences of osteoporosis by adopting changes in lifestyle in order to reduce risk. If a specific preventative treatment exists, which could be administered to the patient, then information on the benefits of the therapy must be explained to the patient. The advice given should advocate preventative therapy in a manner that is acceptable to the patient and with which the patient is likely to comply. Once in place, the preventative treatment must be reviewed on a regular basis to ascertain compliance, acceptability and efficacy. Should the clinical picture of preventing osteoporosis be suspected of change, which would require treatment or further prevention, then referral for investigation would become necessary to ensure that effective clinical management is maintained.

From this it is evident that the screening process is multi-layered; at each stage, a group of people is selected, highlighting the fact that they are at risk of osteoporosis and that intervention is required to change the possible outcome. This stresses that it is important to draw up an optimum programme, targeting resources at those people most in need of their application. The screening programme will require further refining to enable all health professionals to take advantage of lessons learnt from application of screening, which may elicit as yet unsuspected results. Because osteoporosis is a multi-faceted condition it is difficult to isolate those people at greatest risk; at the same time it is clear that implementing such a scheme could result in several different outcomes, such as delaying the onset of the condition until later life, preventing some of the more severe symptoms of the disease or improving the general quality of life.

Improving the application of known preventative and active treatments may well lead to alteration in the course of the condition, giving rise to other complications of the disease and having a bearing on the medication employed. This may lead to greater awareness and better perception of the natural progression of the disease and result in more effective preventative measures and active treatments, stemming from the ongoing research on ways of preserving bone structure and strength.[9]

Indications for treatment

In order to achieve the good standard of care to which the clinical management is committed, it is necessary to state exactly at which point of the disease each treatment option should be given. This is dependent on the patients obtaining, within a reasonable period of time, a referral for bone density measurement by a DEXA scanner in order to determine which treatment will produce the best results.

The necessity for treatment depends on the likelihood of the patient suffering a fracture and all treatment is aimed at reducing this risk. Therefore patients will often be separated into categories of fracture risk from 'low risk' to 'very high risk'. At low risk, the possibility of fracture is negligible – this is deemed normal. The only action is to advise the individual on lifestyle factors in order to prevent problems from arising in the future. The next degree of severity is the first signs of softening of the bone, known as osteopenia, which can be identified from planar X-rays. The action necessary is to give advice on lifestyle changes and administer replacement therapy, in the form of HRT for women and cyclical etidronate for men, together with calcium and vitamin D supplementation where required. The next stage is a confirmed diagnosis of osteoporosis either from signs and symptoms or as is apparent from the bone density measurement shown in the results obtained from a DEXA scanner. Patients with this degree of the condition are at high risk of a fracture and require active treatment with HRT and/or bisphos-phonates (depending on the sex of the patient), supplementation with calcium and vitamin D, together with lifestyle advice. Patients showing the highest level of severity of the condition are at greatest risk of fracture and will have established osteoporosis apparent from previous fractures. They will require all the active treatments listed under high-risk patients, with supportive care for pain control.[9]

Opportunities for screening

In the absence of a national screening programme in the UK, it is impera-tive to make the most of any opportunities arising when patients present with either symptoms of osteoporosis or evidence is gained of a group of patients at high risk of osteoporosis (see Screening Focus, below). The presentation could be at a number of instances within the health com-munity, so it is essential that all health sectors are aware of how to respond to such patients and have procedures in place for directing them to treatment or to referral for further investigation. There is a need for collaborative work across the health care network and a two-way traffic to proffer advice and treatment from primary to secondary care unless direct referrals to services are available.[10]

Patients may be identified from a single presentation, as in the case of a patient suffering from a low-impact facture, which is a clear indi-cation of established osteoporosis. This type of patient would present initially at a hospital accident and emergency department when the injury happened, but would obtain follow-up treatment at a fracture

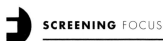

SCREENING FOCUS

Patient groups requiring screening
Low-impact fracture patients
Hysterectomised women
Corticosteroid users
Patients with thyroid conditions
The elderly – women over 65 and men over 75

clinic where the connection between the fracture and osteoporosis should be made. The fracture clinic could be designed to look for these types of fractures associated with osteoporosis and to diagnose or, if uncertain, either perform a DEXA scan or refer for a scan at a later date. At this point, treatment should be commenced by the fracture clinic or the patient should be referred back to their GP to discuss their individual choice of therapy options.

Women who have had a premature menopause following surgical removal of the uterus and ovaries will automatically be given replacement sex hormones, but at the same time should be warned of the possibility of osteoporosis if the hormonal therapy is stopped. These patients need to be followed up, not only because they are on HRT, which can affect blood pressure and clotting, but also because of the possibility of osteoporosis. Advice should be given on lifestyle factors and maintaining a balanced diet with sufficient calcium and vitamin D. This may need to be followed up in a number of years time to check that the hormonal therapy is continuing to prevent osteoporosis and to decide whether it is necessary either to change to alternative therapy or to add in other treatments. In order to make the decision, the patient will need to have further investigations to measure the bone mass density to confirm the requirement for treatment.

Another group of patients who should be monitored are those who have to take corticosteroids for long periods as a result of chronic disease. The ailments from which these patients suffer could be an indicator as to how they could be identified, as they often have to attend review clinics based at either a hospital or general practice surgery. Such patients will be suffering from asthma, rheumatoid arthritis or chronic skin conditions, such as psoriasis. The presence or otherwise of osteoporosis should be considered at the commencement of corticosteroid therapy. Patients should be counselled on lifestyle factors and if a high dose of corticosteroid is to be administered, it may well be that preventative therapy will become necessary. The dose of the corticosteroid should be reviewed on a regular basis and if there is the possibility of stopping the steroid therapy for even a short period this should be encouraged. The move towards the use of short courses of corticosteroids for acute exacerbations of the chronic condition should be standard practice; lower dose maintenance therapy should only be used as a last resort. Patients who have been heavy users of corticosteroids in the past will require to be reviewed not only to reduce the dose if possible, but also to identify the possibility of the presence of osteoporosis and whether it warrants further investigation. Preventative treatment should be given as a matter of course.[11,12]

Patients who have a thyroid condition – either hyperthyroid or hypothyroid – should be targeted, as these conditions affect the regulation of calcium within the body and have a direct bearing on the formation and regulation of bone. This is a particular problem in later life as hypothyroidism and osteoporosis can develop together or precipitate one another. These patients should be monitored closely and a thyroid function test should be carried out on a regular basis to ensure that the correct replacement dose of levothyroxine (thyroxine) is given to prevent the disease and the associated conditions.[13]

Treatment choices

The most expensive drugs are those that are not effective in treating or preventing a disease nor in achieving the desired outcomes. This could be because the therapy in question has been prescribed inappropriately and leads to unwanted side-effects with poor compliance. It is therefore important that therapy is chosen in relationship to the extent of the disease and the ability of the patient to comply with the treatment regimen.

In order to make the most cost-effective use of medications for osteoporosis it is important to have clear information on the choice of drugs, when they are to be used and which is the first choice therapy. The Department of Health should produce clear guidance as to which patient should receive which drug, dependent on the stage of the disease and the requirements of the patient. The guidance should be based on the particular type of osteoporosis seen in an area, how it presents for treatment and the likelihood of the patient complying with the drug treatment. There is a need to continually monitor these patients, as the drug treatment may have to be changed or added to if the required improvement in bone mass is not seen.[3]

Clinical audit

To ensure that a screening programme is working for a particular community, it is essential that a system of analysis is formulated to monitor the effectiveness of the scheme. The major outcomes of the screening programme will involve a number of parameters to be certain that the correct people are targeted. To compound the success of the screening programme, the ensuing investigations should produce a high degree of positive results as only a small portion of the population are benefiting from the process. The most important factor is the reduction in the number of fractures of the hip, spine and wrist, although often only the fractures of the hip and spine are recorded in total and associated with osteoporosis. It will not be possible to totally eliminate fractures, but there should be a reduction in the total number of fractures experienced by patients and they should occur later in life, with lower morbidity rates and higher maintenance of mobility.

References

1. Advisory Group (Chairman: D Barlow). *Report on Osteoporosis*. London: Department of Health, 1994.
2. UK Department of Health. *Strategy for Osteoporosis*. London: Department of Health, 1998.
3. Royal College of Physicians. *Osteoporosis. Clinical Guidelines for Prevention and Treatment*. London: Royal College of Physicians, 1999.
4. South African Medical Association – Osteoporosis Working Group. Osteoporosis clinical guideline. *S Afr Med J* 2000; **90**: 907–944.
5. National Osteoporosis Society. An osteoporosis framework – examples of selective case finding. www.nos.org.uk (accessed 2000).
6. Miller P, McClung M. Prediction of fracture risk I: Bone density. *Am J Med Sci* 1996; **312**: 257–259.
7. Deal C L. Osteoporosis: prevention, diagnosis and management. *Am J Med* 1997; **102**(1A Suppl): 35S–39S.
8. Weinstein L, Ullery B. Identification of at risk women for osteoporosis screening. *Am J Obstet Gynecol* 2000; **183**: 547–549.
9. UK Department of Health. *Quick Reference Primary Care Guide on the Prevention and Treatment of Osteoporosis*. London: Department of Health, 1998.
10. Shah S. Barnet pharmacists advise on effects of diet and medicines on osteoporosis. *Pharm J* 2002; **269**: 801.
11. Walsh L J. Use of oral corticosteroids in the community and the prevention of secondary osteoporosis: a cross sectional study. *BMJ* 1996; **313**: 344–346.
12. O'Donnell L, Holden J. Audit steroid use to limit bone loss. *Health and Ageing* February 2002: 23.
13. National Service Framework (NSF). *Older People*. London: Department of Health, 2001: Standard six: 76–89.

13

Pharmaceutical care of the osteoporotic patient

Pharmaceutical care

When the term 'pharmaceutical care' was first coined, in 1975, it was used in an attempt to define a patient-focused approach that sought to rationalise drug usage whilst limiting possible detrimental effects, such as adverse drug reactions. This described the basic role of the pharmacist at the time, which was to ensure that the correct drug was given to the patient at the right time, whilst being mindful of the needs of the patient. Since this definition was first mooted, the pharmacist's role has developed from merely supplying the drug, to include targeting drug therapy to the specific clinical needs of the patient. These changes mean that the pharmacist is increasingly called upon to advise patients on a one-to-one basis, although until recently no moves had been put in place to monitor the effect that that advice would have on the patient's care and quality of life.[1,2]

Following this evolution of the pharmacist's function within the health system, the definition of pharmaceutical care clearly needed to be updated in order to more accurately reflect the progress that had been made. Hence, in 1990 Hepler and Strand redefined pharmaceutical care into what is acknowledged to be a stance that more closely resembles the status of the pharmacy profession and allows for future development. There is a change of emphasis from drug delivery to the involvement in improvement of patient care and the definition is now worded as follows:[3] 'Pharmaceutical care is defined as the responsible provision of drug therapy for the purpose of achieving definite outcomes that improve a patient's quality of life.'

This definition is now used by pharmacists in a general manner to describe any professional function carried out within the normal working day. In order to develop the parameters involved in pharmaceutical care and to set out in detail the requirements within the term of both the philosophy and the responsibility of the practice, guidance is given on how a practitioner should work. A pharmaceutical care practitioner is defined as a pharmacist who builds up a practice for all the drug-related needs of a patient and who holds him or herself accountable for the meeting of those needs.[4]

Therefore, since the introduction of the concept of pharmaceutical care, the researchers involved have brought about a complete change in direction for the pharmacist, from a role that is mainly product-orientated to one that is orientated to a patient-focused disease process. This moves the pharmacist out of the dispensary into an area of healthcare where patients are seen on an individual basis for review of their medication in the light of their clinical condition. Thus, a practice is built up whereby a pharmacist is associated with a group of patients not necessarily from one therapeutic area, but across a number of clinical conditions where patients are experiencing problems with appropriateness, safety, efficacy and compliance with their prescribed drugs. The practice of pharmaceutical care may now be undertaken in a number of different healthcare settings by either the same practitioner or a network of practitioners in primary and secondary care.[5]

Patients with multiple pathologies will test the skills of the practitioner, as they are more prone to drug-related problems. However, this has not deterred researchers from developing models of practice for a number of specific medical conditions. Whichever model is chosen, this work should be integrated into the current health economy, requiring multidisciplinary working across the care divides. This has been recognised by the International Pharmaceutical Federation as can be seen from the following pronouncement made in 1998:[6]

> Pharmaceutical care is the responsible provision of pharmacotherapy for the purpose of achieving definite outcomes that improve a patient's quality of life. It is a collaborative process that aims to prevent or identify and solve medical product and health related problems. This is a continuous quality improvement process for the use of medicinal products.

The movement towards patient-orientated care establishes a therapeutic relationship between the pharmacist and the patient that can be divided into three stages: (1) assessment, (2) preparation of a care plan, and (3) evaluation (see Pharmaceutical Care Focus below).

PHARMACEUTICAL CARE FOCUS

Elements of pharmaceutical care		
Assessment	*Care plan*	*Evaluation*
Ensure all drug therapy is indicated, effective, safe and convenient	Resolve drug therapy problems	Record actual patient outcomes
Identify drug treatment problems	Achieve therapeutic goals	Evaluate progress in meeting therapeutic goals
	Prevent drug therapy problems	Reassess for new problems

Assessment

This requires identification of all the medication taken by the patient and establishing what is the specific indication for that particular treatment, identifying if it is the safest, most effective and most convenient therapy. Once the need for a drug has been established then any problems arising from the treatment should be solved before moving on to the next phase.

Care plan

The basis of the care plan is the compilation of a complete drug history, with details of previous treatment failures along with current drug therapy. The documentation of these drug-related events should then pave the way for the achievement of the known therapeutic goals stemming from the knowledge of the efficacy of the drug therapy and the normal prognosis of the condition being treated. Once awareness of drug-induced side-effects and the patient's ability to tolerate these has been taken into account, then the care plan can be drawn up, setting out what can be accomplished and how the patient is required to be monitored and followed up.

Evaluation

In the monitoring of the patient, the actual outcomes must be recorded as part of a progress report, which serves as a continuous process so that the care plan can be modified according to the results. At each stage of the evaluation the health of the patient is compared to the therapeutic goals set down in the care plan; these goals may need to be changed in accordance with the known response to treatment. Equally, there is a requirement to ensure that earlier problems have been eradicated; but in all probability, there will be new problems arising, for which new solutions will have to sought.

The structure that pharmaceutical care brings to the practice of clinical pharmacy can be applied to a number of situations; therefore, there is a need for good record keeping which is flexible enough to be of use in different care settings. The model for adoption of a particular programme of pharmaceutical care requires that it links with other health professionals' assessments, care plans and evaluations, complementing and adding to a patient's health record.

Pharmaceutical care in osteoporosis

Having defined and given examples of how pharmaceutical care should be applied, let us now look at its use in the care of preventing and treating osteoporosis and the complications of therapy. In order to do this, various aspects of the condition need to be studied in detail to tease out areas of practice that can be brought to bear to influence the progress of the disease and limit the complications.

The application of pharmaceutical care to osteoporosis will vary depending on the condition of the patient and whether they are suffering from other associated diseases, which could influence the prognosis. Thus, it would be appropriate to divide osteoporosis into a number of stages in order to highlight possible problems (see Pharmaceutical Care Focus, below).[7]

Health promotion

Health promotion should be aimed at all sectors of the population, giving general advice on ways of preventing the likelihood of osteoporosis developing in later life. One section of the population to benefit most from the targeting of this information is teenagers and young people, as they have reached the crucial point in their life where they can do most to build up bone mass and bone strength. Information should also be directed towards the mothers of young children, so that they can reinforce basic messages on diet and exercise to their children as they grow up. Since this advice is based on diet and exercise, the

PHARMACEUTICAL CARE FOCUS

Pharmaceutical care in the prevention and treatment of osteoporosis

---

Health promotion – general information on prevention to all sectors of the population

General prevention – aim at older people who are at greatest risk

Preventative treatments – given to patients at risk of fractures due to osteoporosis

Active treatment – medication given to actively promote bone mass gain

Treating active disease – treatment of the complications of osteoporotic fractures

---

mother is usually the person in the family best placed to supervise the implementation of appropriate measures.

There are a number of ways to ensure that the information is available to the target audience. For example, leaflets and posters can be displayed in community pharmacies, doctors' surgeries, hospital out-patient clinics, especially those dealing with paediatrics and antenatal conditions, schools, sport's facilities and community centres. The health promotion should be designed in such a way as to encourage good practices in children, especially through the teenage years by motivating them to continue with good habits.

General prevention

General preventative measures include advice aimed mainly at the adult population. This can range from the straightforward health promotion messages given earlier to more specific material emphasising the importance of restraint from negative lifestyle factors such as smoking and drinking alcohol to excess. This type of information could be issued as a general directive within a healthy living programme, especially if that includes advice on smoking cessation and knowing your limit of alcohol intake.

A specific group of people to benefit from advice would be those suffering from an underlying disease that could lead to osteoporosis in later life, particularly if the disease concerned is preventable with treatment. This includes young women who have menstrual disorders giving rise to amenorrhoea, which can lead to osteoporosis early in life because of loss of bone following from low levels of oestrogen. Such menstrual problems can result from eating disorders, in which a woman may reduce her dietary intake to a level where the body ceases to menstruate in order to conserve body protein. Amenorrhoea can also occur in women who take a high level of exercise but fail to increase their food intake in order to compensate for high energy needs.

Women who are approaching the menopause should be advised of the possibility of suffering from osteoporosis; at this stage, information should be given regarding hormone replacement therapy (HRT). There are a few contraindications to HRT, namely previous thromboembolic disease and pre-existing cardiac disease. Although women with these conditions will be unable to receive replacement therapy, they can be given alternative therapy to reduce the symptoms of the menopause and for the long-term prevention of osteoporosis if it is thought they are at high risk. If a woman decides that HRT is an option to be considered then this must be reviewed in the light of current therapy and any other conditions she may have, together with reference to evidence from the family history. All these factors should be assessed prior to deciding which HRT product would be most appropriate for a particular woman. If a woman has had previous breast cancer or has a family history of breast cancer, then routine HRT may not be wise and the selective oestrogen receptor modulator raloxifene would be a better choice, as it should not affect tumour growth.

HRT is frequently associated with nausea along with other related gastrointestinal problems, which could be reduced by the use of a lower dose, transdermal or patch presentation. Skin problems can occur, particularly the appearance of irregular brown macules or freckles on the face. HRT can elevate the blood pressure; therefore prior to commencement of HRT and during treatment the blood pressure should be monitored on a regular basis because if the blood pressure rises enough to warrant a diagnosis of hypertension then the therapy should be stopped at once. A further reason for cessation of HRT would be tests showing abnormal liver function, especially if jaundice were present and the patient had a past history of such abnormality.

The major problem for women on HRT is the return of menstrual bleeding. This can be eliminated by using continuous combined therapy, which will improve patient compliance with the treatment. There are several drug interactions, mainly involving the oestrogen ingredient of the combined replacement therapy. Enzyme inducers such as rifampicin, phenytoin and carbamazepine can reduce the effect of the oestrogen by speeding up the metabolism. Oestrogen itself can enhance the effects of some of the corticosteroids by decreasing the hepatic metabolism of these drugs, leading to higher blood levels for longer periods.

HRT comes in a number of different dosage preparations, regimens and pharmaceutical forms to enable patients to tolerate the medication and to remember when to take or apply the next dose. A woman who feels that she already takes enough medication, may benefit from a once-a-week preparation rather than a daily dosage regimen.

Another at-risk group are patients with either hyperthyroidism or hypothyroidism, as both these conditions interfere with calcium uptake into the bone and may lead to inefficient bone production with a consequential reduction in bone mass. In order to prevent these problems from arising it is important to maintain the thyroid function test result within the normal range and to correct any hypocalcaemia. Similarly, in patients with kidney or liver disease, problems may arise in the metabolism and activation of vitamin D. This is normally prevented by prescribing supplements and correction of the calcium level. Patients with any of these conditions should be made aware that the long-term consequence of not 'getting it right' is the onset of osteoporosis.

In later life, our ability to obtain both calcium and vitamin D directly from the diet and the environment declines, making it important that supplements of these essential nutrients are taken to maintain body functions – in this case for bone remodelling. In later life people should be considered for supplementation with calcium and vitamin D to maintain bone function and bone mass.

Preventative treatments

There will be patients who, for a number of reasons, are at risk of developing osteoporosis if preventative measures are not instigated. They may even have a mild form of the disease and require preventative therapy to slow down progression, with the emphasis on preventing the long-term effects such as fractures.

The first group of people are women in whom a premature surgical or natural menopause has occurred. These women will require long-term HRT, if not contraindicated. Additional therapy such as bisphosphonates may be necessary if the effectiveness of HRT reduces with time or if complications occur. These patients will need close monitoring in order to prevent bone mass reducing to such an extent that the risk of fracture is high. Knowledge of bone mass in these people will be crucial, as this will change the clinical management of the condition.

Similarly, patients who have been treated for long-term hypothyroidism may need to take calcium and vitamin D supplementation to prevent the possibility of low levels of calcium. It may also be wise to investigate further to discover if there are any signs of early osteoporosis, which will require additional treatment.

The largest group in need of close monitoring are those patients who have been taking large doses of oral corticosteroids because of long-term autoimmune disease. A careful selection of these patients should be undertaken giving regard to previous records of drug treatment and the length of time since diagnosis with the related disease. The critical factor is the number of months during which a patient receives in excess of the equivalent of 7.5 mg of prednisolone; this will determine the degree of bone mass loss. If the time period of corticosteroid use has been greater than six months at a high dosage, there is a strong likelihood of excessive bone mass loss, and preventative treatment will be required. If a patient has been taking corticosteroids for 3–6 months they will need to be investigated to establish that no other risk factors exist, otherwise prevention should be offered. Patients who have been on corticosteroid therapy for less than three months should be monitored further and given advice on prevention with the proviso that there could be a future need to consider preventative treatment.

Corticosteroid treatment is normally prescribed for conditions such as rheumatoid arthritis, asthma, chronic obstructive pulmonary disease (COPD), chronic skin diseases, haematological disorders, chronic gastrointestinal diseases and, as an adjunct, some cancers. Thus there are several different groups of patients taking corticosteroids and these will need to be assessed initially to find out whether they are at risk of osteoporosis and prevention given if necessary. Thereafter, new patients should be advised of the long-term problems and how they can be prevented, and that in the future preventative drug treatment may be essential because of their underlying condition.

Active treatment

Active treatment will be required for patients who have been diagnosed as having osteoporosis either through diagnostic tests or because they fit into a known at-risk category and have shown preliminary signs and symptoms. The treatment will include a bisphosphonate in conjunction with adequate doses of calcium and vitamin D or, if indicated, HRT.

These patients will have to be able to tolerate the bisphosphonates, which must be taken on an empty stomach. In some cases this means not eating food either two hours before or two hours after taking the medication. Bisphosphonates cause upper gastrointestinal irritation in a significant proportion of patients; this occurs even when the medication is taken with a large volume of water and the patient stands upright. To overcome this problem two of the drugs have been formulated into a 'once-a-week' preparation, which limits the discomfort and the need to abstain from food to just one day a week. The once-a-week preparation is also beneficial for patients who are already taking a number of other medications and have difficulty in ensuring that certain tablets are not taken together.

For patients with established osteoporosis who have not yet sustained any fractures, the most positive course of action is to reduce the risk of fracture by reducing the likelihood of a fall. For instance within pharmaceutical care, there are a number of drugs that cause drowsiness, dizziness or postural hypotension; all medication that could cause the osteoporotic patient to experience these effects should be reviewed in order to reduce the risk of the patient falling and sustaining a fracture. Drugs to be discontinued or eliminated if possible include the hypnotics, which have a hangover effect on the following day, and other drugs that can cause drowsiness, such as the older antidepressants and antipsychotics. If this type of drug is necessary to the patient's well-being, then a substitution of one of the newer agents, with less or little associated sedation should be made. The problem of postural hypotension can arise when antihypertensive therapy is first administered. It may persist until the body adjusts to the lower blood pressure, but if the symptoms continue the chosen drug should be reviewed with the aim of finding a drug that is better tolerated.

Treating active disease

Patients who have already had a fracture as a result of osteoporosis will require all the treatments and assessments that can be offered to patients in the active treatment group above. They should have experienced a programme of rationalisation of their drug therapy to limit problems without suffering any detrimental effect on their quality of life. The difference between the active disease group patients and the active treatment group patients is that the former will have already suffered a wrist, hip or vertebral fracture, which requires additional management strategies.

In the instance of a wrist or colles fracture, the patient will require analgesia to reduce the associated pain and to help in the healing of the fracture. The analgesia will be given for a short period while the fracture heals, therefore the use of short-term nonsteroidal anti-inflammatories (NSAIDs) or strong analgesics may be necessary without affecting other long-term therapy.

A hip fracture requires immediate medical help and admission to hospital for repair and either prosthetic replacement of support of the bone or replacement of the joint, depending on the extent of the damage incurred during the fracture. This will require strong analgesia while the patient rehabilitates, with particular emphasis on mobilisation. The medication prescribed will concentrate on enabling the patient to endure movement and allowing rehabilitation to progress, otherwise delays could lengthen the healing process and lead to further complications. Once the patient is able to cope independently with the activities of daily life, the analgesia can be reduced and used only when the patient is going to be engaged in any activity likely to produce pain. Although a short course of NSAIDs may be required postoperatively, this should not be continued on a longer term basis as greater damage may be inflicted on the existing bone because of bone mass loss. Strong analgesics can be sedating when used for a short period but when given over an extended length of time these side-effects should diminish in due course.

The fracture that poses most problems in both detection and treatment is the vertebral fracture. Problems arise if the initial pain is not severe and tapers off later after a day or two. The link between back pain and osteoporosis is one that is not immediately made, and the connection may only be apparent if the patient is questioned on risk factors such as details of family history, lifestyle and current drug therapy. Once the cause of the fracture has been isolated, treatment can be given to prevent further damage and to actively treat the osteoporosis.

One of the dangers of the vertebral fracture in osteoporosis is that fragmentation of the broken bone may occur, causing pain varying in severity from mild intermittent to very severe, especially if a fragment of bone puts pressure on a nerve. This can cause a sharp, shooting pain that even strong analgesics may fail to counteract. A patient may also experience a series of short sharp pains caused by pressure from several loose fragments of splintered bone, adding to the difficulty in treating this type of fracture. The severity of the pain can alter drastically in a short space of time. Analgesia plays a secondary role in controlling pain while investigations are undertaken, and surgery may be necessary to remove bone fragments and prevent further damage. If surgery is not carried out, analgesia may be required for a number of years in increasing amounts, which may result in a number of combination preparations being used. Often, a strong analgesic such as codeine or dihydrocodeine given in maximum doses is required to eliminate the pain. The use of lower doses in combination preparations such as co-dydramol and co-codamol may well leave the patient in pain, and if in order to produce a satisfactory result the maximum dose of the combination product has to be exceeded, then this can lead to complications in the form of side-effects. If the patient suffers pressure on a nerve, then antiepileptics and some of the tricyclic antidepressants such as amitriptyline may offer relief.

Pharmaceutical care projects

A pharmaceutical care project entails the preparation of a complete strategy for areas in which the pharmacist and other health professionals can be brought together to produce a complete pharmaceutical care programme. As yet, the format has not been produced in respect of osteoporosis, although there are proposals for such schemes for asthma, diabetes, angina, hypertension and hyperlipidaemia. There are, however, reports of projects that are related to the identification of osteoporosis and the use of assessments to promote prevention (see Pharmaceutical Care Focus, below).

Falls project

This is a project run by a group of community pharmacists who instigated this work in the communities of older people across a number of health authorities. Celebrities were employed to publicise the role of the pharmacist and to demonstrate how help and advice could be obtained on aspects of healthcare, mainly related to the prevention of falls.

PHARMACEUTICAL CARE FOCUS

Pharmaceutical care projects in prevention and treatment of osteoporosis

Falls project – evaluation of the associated risks of falling in patients at risk of osteoporosis

Osteoporosis screening at a community pharmacy – a survey of people at risk of osteoporosis with direct referral for diagnostic tests

Audit of corticosteroid use – primary care evaluation of corticosteroid use in the elderly with a view to prevention of osteoporosis

The project dealt with reviews of the medication of elderly people that were carried out by community pharmacists. These were undertaken to identify those preparations that can contribute to falls. During the course of the review, the pharmacists also gave information on hazards in the home that could contribute to a fall. Dietary advice was given, describing ways of increasing the intake of calcium and vitamin D and the types of physical activity classes available that would involve exercises to maintain both bone mass and bone strength.

This is a good example of a pharmaceutical care approach identifying a specific risk in a group of the population who are prone to osteoporosis. This would be classified as general prevention through advice on drug therapy, the avoidance of hazards and participation in beneficial physical exercises, while following a healthy diet.[8]

Osteoporosis screening

In a pilot scheme operated in a community pharmacy, patients over the age of 60 entering the community pharmacy were asked whether they would be willing to participate. First they filled in a questionnaire, then they were offered a bone mineral density scan using a dual-energy X-ray absorptiometry (DEXA) scanner. The degree of risk was assessed from the number of criteria they fulfilled according to the questionnaire. The bone mineral density scan was carried out on the patient's heel by the nurse. People who were thought to have osteoporosis, based on the questionnaire results and bone density measurement, were immediately referred to their general practitioner. Those found to be at increased risk of osteoporosis were given information on bone health and advised to consult their general practitioner in the near future.

In the next phase of the project, a trained pharmacist will be responsible for prescribing medication under the auspices of a patient group direction. This project is an example of a preventative treatment strategy, whereby patients thought to be at risk of osteoporosis are actively identified through completing a risk assessment questionnaire.[9]

Corticosteroid drug use

A general practitioner who was mindful of the need to comply with the National Service Framework (NSF) for elderly people, which directs that such patients should have their medication regularly reviewed, decided to carry out a survey of all elderly patients in his practice who could be at risk of osteoporosis based on a case finding strategy. Patients who had been prescribed or were regularly taking corticosteroids in excess of the equivalent of prednisolone 7.5 mg for a period greater than six months and those who had been given a cumulative dose greater than 1 g were identified by means of a computer search of the practice list and were offered a DEXA scan. Any such patients who were diagnosed as having osteoporosis were given blood tests to confirm the results. Then the doctor instituted preventative treatment to attempt to arrest the progression to established osteoporosis. It is proposed to review the situation in six months' time to investigate how these patients have fared in the light of the medical intervention and to discover what degree of success, if any, has been achieved.

This example illustrates how preventative measures can be used to treat a section of the population who display numerous risk factors for osteoporosis, namely old age, underlying associated pathology and the use of corticosteroids. This action was taken as a fundamental measure in the NSF for elderly people and should be commended and publicised as good practice so that other general practitioners and health authorities take note and evaluate the action. It need not be left to general practitioners working on their own, as it is often customary for a pharmacist to advise on medication reviews to be undertaken in respect of certain groups of patients who are receiving repeat prescriptions.[10,11]

Although these pharmaceutical care projects are encouraging and are attempting to tackle problems associated with drug use, both in the treatment of osteoporosis and in the drug induction of osteoporosis, they are still in their infancy. It is hoped that, building on work commenced in a pilot project, further funding will be provided to expand progression into a full-scale working model. These projects are investigating only one aspect of the problem, involving a minimum number of health professions. In order to make them work more effectively and widen the spectrum there must be more collaboration between health professionals across all disciplines and sectors of the health service.

References

1. Mikeal R L, Brown T P, Lazarus H L, *et al.* Quality of pharmaceutical care in hospitals. *Am J Hosp Pharm* 1975; **3**: 567–574.
2. Crown report. *Review of prescribing, supply and administration of medicines.* London: Department of Health, 1999.
3. Hepler C, Strand L, Opportunities and responsibilities in pharmaceutical care. *Am J Hosp Pharm* 1990; **47**: 533–543.
4. Cippole R, Strand L. Challenges in pharmaceutical care. *Am J Hosp Pharm* 1993; **50**: 1618–1621.

5. Posey L M, Pharmaceutical care: will pharmacy incorporate its philosophy of practice. *J Am Pharm Assoc* 1997; **NS37**: 145–148.
6. International Pharmaceutical Federation. Statement on pharmaceutical care. www.fip.nl/pdf/pharmcare/pdf (accessed July 2002).
7. National Osteoporosis Society. An osteoporosis framework – meeting health needs. www.nos.org.uk (accessed 2000).
8. Long R, Black J. How pharmacists can make a difference in managing osteoporosis and falls. *Pharm J* 2002; **269**: 534.
9. Patel H. A community pharmacy run screening programme for osteoporosis. *Pharm J* 2002; **268**: 419.
10. Cooper A. GP strategy helps PCG deliver NSF standards on osteoporosis. *Guidelines in Practice* 2001; **4**(12): 25–30.
11. National Service Framework (NSF). *Older People.* London: Department of Health, 2001: Standard six: 76–89.

Glossary

Achlorhydria Condition caused by a failure of the stomach to produce hydrochloric acid, creating either a neutral or an alkaline environment in the stomach. Can affect the digestion of food, causing absorption problems with essential nutrients.

Adipose tissue A fibrous connective tissue packed with fat cells. It forms a thick layer under the skin, mainly around the kidneys and buttocks, providing an insulating layer and an energy store.

Alcopop An alcoholic drink with a high sugar content and a strong, sweet flavour to disguise the presence of the alcohol. Similar in taste to many so-called soft or non-alcoholic drinks.

Alfacalcidol A form of vitamin D that has undergone hydroxylation in the kidney. Frequently administered to patients suffering significantly impaired renal function in order to overcome the lack of natural hydroxylation. Can be given by mouth or in severe cases by an intravenous injection. Calcium blood levels should be monitored during therapy to prevent hypercalcaemia.

Anabolic steroids Agents promoting metabolism involved in protein synthesis in cells, leading to tissue growth. Often used to produce weight gain in the frail or to improve bone marrow cell synthesis in seriously ill patients. Based on male sex hormones, anabolic steroids will promote male secondary sexual characteristics in women.

Androgens A group of steroid sex hormones, including testosterone and androsterone, responsible for masculinisation. Produced naturally in the male, these hormones are prescribed to patients suffering deficiency disease or in cases of delayed puberty.

Biochemical markers Biochemical substances that, when subjected to certain tests, can indicate by a serum level the cause of a problem. For example, for osteoporosis the biochemical markers are calcium, phosphate and vitamin D.

Bone formation   The process whereby bone is created from the raw materials. It involves the uptake of calcium into cartilage tissue causing the cartilage to become rigid due to mineralisation.

Bone Gla protein   A protein fundamental to the production of the architecture of bone providing the strength. It can be measured as an indication of bone formation.

Bone matrix   A network of cartilage tissue that is formed before the growth of the bone. Calcium is deposited within the matrix by mineralisation, producing a rigid structure prior to the formation of new bone.

Bone mineral density   A measurement of the ability of bone to alter a single beam of radiation over a defined length of bone or two beams of radiation produced from two different sources. From this capacity to absorb radiation, the density of the bone can be calculated and quoted as a value on a scale, which is compared with a standard.

Bone multicellular unit   A unit of bone that is capable of undergoing remodelling.

Calcar femorale   A spur-like projection from the femoral bone of the thigh, which helps to strengthen the neck of the femur.

Calcitriol   An analogue of vitamin D which has been hydrolysed; it therefore requires no further metabolism, either in the liver or the kidney, before becoming active.

Canaliculi   A small channel or canal seen in compact bone, linking lacunae containing bone cells.

Cancellous bone   A lattice-like structure, present in bone as part of its development. Also seen as part of the consolidation stage of a fracture repair. A structure within mature bone, which has low density and is surrounded by the denser cortical bone.

Chelation   The process whereby certain chemical compounds bind metal ions causing these to become inert. If this occurs within the gastrointestinal tract the chelation will reduce or prevent absorption of the metal ion.

Cisternae   Large spaces present in the bone; these act as a reservoir aiding the drainage of fluid from the thoracic bones into the lymph glands.

Colles fracture A fracture of the lower end of the radius and the tip of the ulna just above the wrist. Usually sustained when the hand is outstretched to arrest the action of a fall.

Committee on Safety of Medicines (CSM) An independent body which reviews the reporting of adverse drug reactions in the UK, producing bulletins to inform prescribers of the side-effects associated with particular drugs.

Cortical bone The outer layer of bone; it is a compact and solid tissue comprising bone tissue laid down in circular layers.

Cushing's syndrome A condition caused by excessive amounts of corticosteroids in the body, arising either from overactivity of the adrenal glands or from a prolonged period of intake of doses of corticosteroid larger than physiological doses.

Cytokines Proteins released by cells as a result of an antigen reaction through which they communicate with other cells via receptors.

Demineralisation The process whereby minerals are released from bone as part of the bone remodelling function. N.B. Excessive elimination of inorganic salts causes osteomalacia.

Fissure fracture A fracture of the bone, manifesting as a crack, most commonly found in the skull.

Fluoride A compound of fluorine, commonly added to the water supply to reduce dental caries in children. Actively given as a treatment for osteoporosis because it combines with bone tissue to improve bone mineral density.

Fracture risk The estimated risk of contracting a fracture based on the bone mineral density and previous fracture history.

Fracture neck of femur A fracture occurring at the point at which the femur is angled into the pelvis forming the hip joint. Commonly seen in elderly patients with osteoporosis who have sustained a fall.

Free radicals An atom or group of atoms possessing an odd electron, causing the resulting atom or atoms to become highly reactive with any surrounding tissue as it attempts to pair off the free electron.

Glycoproteins A group of compounds consisting of a protein and a carbohydrate, these compounds can be enzymes, hormones or antigens.

Golgi bodies/apparatus   A collection of vesicles and folded membranes used to store and transport secretions manufactured by the endoplasmic reticulum in secretory cells.

Haversian canals/system   A cylindrical unit of which compact bone is made, which forms a central tube surrounded by bone matrix and bone cells linked by smaller channels or canals.

High-density lipoproteins   A group of proteins found in the blood plasma and lymph, and combined with fat into the membranes of cells.

Hip protectors   Foam padding in the form of an undergarment, worn over the hip to reduce the impact of a fall on the hip bone, thus preventing a fracture neck of femur.

Hormone replacement therapy (HRT)   A term used to define the supplementation of any natural hormone. When prescribed for osteoporosis it refers to the replacement of oestrogen and progestogen.

Howship's lacunae   A small cavity that functions as a channel of absorption.

Hydroxyapatite   An inorganic compound (a complex form of calcium phosphate) which gives rigidity to bone and teeth.

Hypercalciuria   An abnormally high concentration of calcium in the urine.

Lacuna   A small cavity or depression, a space within compact bone in which the bone cell lies.

Lamellae   In bone, thin layers of calcified matrix surrounding Haversian canals in a circular pattern.

Leukocyte   Commonly known as a white blood cell, may be further defined as a blood cell with a nucleus and cell contents, or a blood cell without haemoglobin. Divided into different classes based on function and appearance.

Low-density lipoproteins   A group of proteins found in blood plasma and lymph, combined with fat and used to transport lipids throughout the body.

Mastocytoma   A benign tumour of a mast cell made up of a numerous mast cells, forming a nodulous tumour.

Menopause   The period in a woman's life when she ceases to produce egg cells from her ovaries and stops menstruating. Levels of oestrogen and progestogen fall dramatically, producing a number of related symptoms.

Mineralisation   The process whereby calcium is deposited into cartilage and converted into bone material.

National Osteoporosis Society   A UK self-help group for people with osteoporosis, which promotes health awareness and the prevention of osteoporosis to the general public and informs health professionals about evidence for treatment protocols and production of advice to patients.

Ossification   A three-stage process bought about by the osteoblasts that results in the formation of bone. The overall effect is that cartilage tissue is converted into bone.

Osteomalacia   A softening of bone caused by a lack of vitamin D, which leads to a reduction in the calcium content of the bone.

Osteopenia   Loss of bone mass below normal level due to insufficient bone synthesis.

Paget's disease   Also known as osteitis deformans, a chronic disease of bone, in which the bones of the skull, limbs and spine become thick and soft. Often associated with pain.

Peak bone mass   The maximum bone mass of an individual, attained from the mid-twenties to the early thirties at the latest. Greater in men than in women.

Prostacyclin   A transmitter substance, often released at site of injury, rousing the inflammatory response and the cause of pain.

Rickets   A disease of childhood, characterised by a softening of bones resulting in deformities of the long bones. The cause of this condition is poor nutrition, leading to lack of vitamin D and calcium.

Salcatonin   A source of calcitonin derived from salmon used in supplementation and in the treatment of hypercalcaemia and Paget's disease.

Sciatica   Pain felt in the back and often down the leg, usually caused by an intervertebral disc breaking down, producing a sideways protrusion onto a spinal nerve.

Selective serotonin reuptake inhibitors A group of drugs that affect the uptake of serotonin and are used for the treatment of depression.

Somatomedins A protein hormone produced by the liver in response to the effect of growth hormone, promoting protein synthesis and growth.

Spicules Small splinters of bone.

Sterols A group of compounds related to the steroids, the most important is cholesterol.

Trabecular bone The inner core of bone, in the form of thin bars, which provides the strength of the bone.

Tumour necrosis factor Two proteins that function as cytokines and are responsible for the destruction of damaged tissue such as cancer cells.

Recommended reading

Consensus Development Conference; diagnosis, prophylaxis and treatment of osteo-porosis. *Am J Med* 1993; **94**: 646–650.

Francis R M. *Osteoporosis: Pathogenesis and Management*. Dordrecht: Kluwer Academic, 1990.

Kanis J A. *Osteoporosis*. Oxford: Blackwell Healthcare Communications, 1997.

Marcus R, Feldman D, Alto P, Kelsey J. *Osteoporosis*. London: Academic Press, 2001.

Royal College of Physicians. *Osteoporosis. Clinical Guidelines for Prevention and Treatment*. London: Royal College of Physicians, 1999.

Sartoris D J. *Osteoporosis: Diagnosis and Treatment*. New York: Marcel Dekker, 1996.

South African Medical Association – Osteoporosis Working Group. Osteoporosis clinical guideline. *S Afr Med J* 2000; **90**: 907–944.

Woolf A D, Dixon A S. *Osteoporosis: a Clinical Guide*. London: Martin Dunitz, 1988.

Index